RECONSTRUCTIVE AESTHETIC IMPLANT SURGERY

RECONSTRUCTIVE AESTHETIC IMPLANT SURGERY

Abd El Salam El Askary

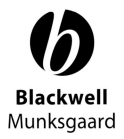

Blackwell
Munksgaard

Published in the U.S. by
Iowa State Press
A Blackwell Publishing Company

© 2003 Blackwell Munksgaard,
Published By Iowa State Press
A Blackwell Publishing Company

Iowa State Press
2121 State Avenue, Ames, Iowa 50014-8300, USA
Tel: +1 515 292 0140
Web site: www.iowastatepress.com

Editorial Offices:
9600 Garsington Road, Oxford OX4 2DQ
Tel: +44 01865 776868

Blackwell Publishing Asia Pty Ltd,
550 Swanston Street, Carlton South,
Victoria 3053, Australia
Tel: +61 (0)3 9347 0300

Blackwell Verlag
Kurfürstendamm 57, 10707 Berlin, Germany
Tel: +49 (0)30 32 79 060

Europe and Asia

Library of Congress Cataloging-in-Publication Data
El Askary, Abd El Salam
  Reconstructive aesthetic implant surgery / Abd El Salam
    El Askary
    p. ; cm.
Includes bibliographical references and index.
  ISBN 0-8138-2108-8
  1. Dental implants. 2. Dental implants—Aesthetic implants.
  [DNLM: 1. Dental Implantation—methods. 2. Reconstructive Surgical Procedures—methods. WU 640 E37r 2003]
  I. Title
  RK667.I45E4 2003
  617.6'92—dc21   2002155992

ISBN: 0-8138-2108-8

Cover art: From the portrait of Irma Brunner by Edouard Manet. © Photo RMN—Jean Schormans; reprinted by permission.

Set in Sabon by D&G Limited, LLC
Printed and bound in Korea by Doosan Printing

For further information on
Blackwell Publishing, visit our website:
www.blackwellpublishing.com
          or
www.iowastatepress.com

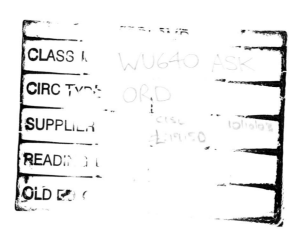

Contents

Foreword

The Kubler Ross emotional progression of anger, denial, despair, bargaining, and finally acceptance when facing serious illnesses or even death applies also to significant loss of teeth and related oral-facial structures. The advances that have been made in implant dentistry allow us to interrupt this downward spiral for many patients and virtually reconstruct their hard and soft tissue deficits.

Originally, implants were devised to restore function, and aesthetics was secondary. Soldiers suffering from the ravages of World War II and later conflicts cried out for effective therapies. Dental implants, devised by multiple clinicians and investigators from around the world, often provided the foundation for functional prostheses.

As the field matured, many cases required a multidisciplinary approach with identification of complex etiologic factors. This central issue was often ignored or not appreciated. Challenges were met with compromise. End goals were not clear. No one or everyone wanted to be the "captain of the ship." An educational revolution with significant cross-training was the result. The upheaval of commitment to excellence is still raging full force.

Today, in order to achieve the aesthetic results that our patients rightfully demand, many foundational cosmetic procedures are now recognized as being necessary. Dr. El Askary's text traces the history of, describes, and illustrates the hard and soft tissue manipulations for optimal results with implant-supported prostheses.

Personally, we both feel that in the arena of "cosmetic dentistry" there is too much emphasis placed on signature cases, tooth preparation, cementation and finishing of veneers, metal-free bridges, etc. and not enough emphasis placed on our ability to create the necessary bone support and gingival architectures that are the sine qua non for aesthetic case outcomes.

Dr. El Askary has confronted these scientific and practical clinical training problems head on. He has given the profession a treatise on how we should proceed when approaching simple as well as definitively complex cases. His work is to be admired in the original meaning of the word, i.e., "wondered at." He is to be congratulated. Our patients need no longer sink to despair.

With our best personal and professional regards, we remain

Sincerely,

Carl E. Misch, DDS, MDS, FACD, FICD
Co-Chairman, ICOI
Beverly Hills, Michigan, USA

Kenneth W.M. Judy, DDS, FACD, FICD
Co-Chairman, ICOI
New York, New York, USA

Preface

In the name of God, the Beneficent, the Merciful.

The fashioning of modern dental implantology in the hands of pioneers like Branemark, Linkow, Judy, Niznick, Straumann, Misch, and others has solved many chronic clinical problems that were heretofore untreatable. Dental implants are becoming sometimes the only predictable alternative treatment for many clinical situations, and their long-term success over time has been well established. New implant designs with improved surgical and prosthodontic options have extended the benefits of implant dentistry to patients previously excluded from therapy due to anatomical limitations or other reasons. Today, countless numbers of patients with partial and full edentulism have experienced dramatic improvements not only in clinical function, but also in their appearance, social interactions, and personal self-confidence as a direct result of successful implant therapy. In that vein, modern dental implantology may be considered the treatment modality of the twentieth century, and it promises to yield even greater advancements in the new millennium.

Concurrent with the refinement of the scientific aspects of dental implants, many renowned clinicians around the world, such as Lazara, Bragger, Potashnick, Hurzeler, Belser, Tarnow, Salama, Bengazi, Sclar, Wohrle, Saadoun, Grunder, Bitchacho, Geovanovick, Kan, Zitzmann, and others, have made invaluable advancements in the science of aesthetic implantology. Through the contributions of these master artists, dentists no longer need to make the painful compromise between providing the patient with function at the expense of appearance, or vice versa. I have greatly benefited from their contributions.

I offer in this present work an overview of the beauty and artistic qualities that may be achieved with dental implants. The surgical and reconstructive aspects of aesthetic dental implant restorations are presented, along with a step-by-step clinical manual to aid practitioners in achieving optimum clinical results.

The first chapter of this book highlights the importance of art in human life and its relation to implant dentistry. It shows how implant dentistry uniquely combines science and art to achieve a functional, aesthetic result. It is worth noting that this field requires not only clinical knowledge but also artistic talent to provide satisfactory results.

The second chapter concentrates on the presurgical planning for aesthetic cases, from evaluations of the study cast to the fabrication of the surgical template. The chapter highlights the available treatment options and explains why one treatment option should be selected over another. It also covers the provisional stage preparation for the patient receiving an implant-supported prosthesis in the aesthetic zone; hence, the chapter focuses on much more than aesthetic case planning.

The third chapter of this book addresses dental implant anatomy, the importance of implant positioning on the alveolar ridge, and how the three-dimensional placement of an implant can be vital to the final treatment outcome. It also addresses the clinical challenges and options for addressing implant misplacements.

The fourth chapter of this book concerns soft tissue management around dental implants. It is the largest chapter of the book and presents most of the soft tissue techniques that are currently available. I have divided the topic into four categories, each of which relates to the timing of clinical intervention. The chapter focuses on many clinical techniques that can be important for the reader and includes guidelines for second-stage surgery, soft tissue grafting, papilla regeneration, and soft tissue enhancement procedures.

The fifth chapter of this book provides information on aesthetic bone reconstruction and presents the methods for grafting the alveolar ridge to attain an optimal aesthetic result. The chapter emphasizes the use of titanium mesh to help solve many clinical problems related to aesthetics and function as a predictable treatment option. It also discusses why certain procedures may be preferable to others, and highlights most of the available bone grafting materials.

It is hoped that the information and clinical techniques included in the present work will provide clinicians with sufficient knowledge to help them achieve aesthetic implant-supported restorations and provide their patients with beauty as one result of the treatment.

Acknowledgments

As instructed by my God to work and provide a quality work as much as possible, because he shall see my work, I thank him first for giving me the strength and inspiring me with vision to write this book.

This book reflects the influences of many mentors and scholars, all of whom I would like to acknowledge personally and offer my debt of gratitude. As for my start in the field of dental implants long ago, I would like to express my profound appreciation for the remarkable educators who guided me with extreme and selfless dedication: Prof. Dr. Roland M. Meffert of San Antonio, Texas, who taught me the A-B-C's and mindset of oral implantology; Prof. Dr. Griffin of Boston, Massachusetts, who showed me the way to soft tissue handling and inspired me as his hands worked with the scalpel during his famous soft tissue grafts; Prof. Dr. Besada of Cleveland, Ohio, who helped me with my unceasing periodontal inquiries; and Prof. Dr. Morton L. Perel of Providence, Rhode Island, who taught me how to provide a publication that is readable! Furthermore, being honored with the ICOI's prestigious Ralph McKinney Award in 1999 had a tremendous impact on my life. I must also acknowledge that the personal advice provided by Dr. Perel and his wife, Jane, was highly valuable in my career.

Other inspiring mentors that I would like to thank are Prof. Dr. Kenneth Judy of New York, who gave me tremendous support, and Prof. Dr. Carl Misch (whom I count as a great scientist and a personal friend). One of the remarkable moments of my life came when Dr. Misch stood up in the conference lecture room in Istanbul, Turkey, after one of my presentations and acknowledged the work that I presented before I even knew him personally. I would also like to acknowledge Prof. Dr. Peker Sandalli, president of the ICOI, and Dr. Eddi Palti, president of the DGZI, who have long supported me by their continuous encouragement.

I must thank my friend and colleague Dr. Luc Huys, who agreed to coauthor the last chapter of this book with me. His efforts were an extreme asset to the book.

I would also like to thank deeply my laboratory technicians, Mr. Walter Lummer (my master technician) and Dr. Raffat Mahfooz for their art work provided in this book. Their contributions have added a great dimension.

I would like to thank the Centerpulse, dental division employees who offered unlimited support for me in the early stages of this book: the maestro of the firm, Mr. Steven Hanson, as well as Celine Cendras-Maret, Robin Marx, and Werner Grotz.

Prosthodontists who helped me along the way by enlightening me with their knowledge were Drs. Abulnaga, El Ibrashi, Sameh Labib, El Sharkawy, Garana, and El Tenneer in Cairo, Egypt.

I must raise my hat and salute the editors who helped me with this book, as I sometimes gave them a hard time (as my first language is Arabic and not English). I would like to thank Mrs. Inas, Dr. Bassant, and Dr. Zahran of Cairo, Egypt, Mrs. Bonnie Harmon of USA and a special thanks goes to my friend Mr. Mike Werner from the Centerpulse dental division team. His dedicated work cannot be forgotten and is highly appreciated.

In the early stages of this book, I collected a large number of articles from the literature and I acknowledge Dr. Racha Fouad of Pennsylvania, Dr. M. Hassan of Boston, Dr. Zaher of Alexandria, and Dr. Thomas Oates of San Antonio for providing scientific materials; without their help this book would not be as it is today.

There were also many friends all over the world who supported the idea of this book wholeheartedly. Thanks to all of you, especially to my personal friends: the famous Arab actress Yosra, my dear friend Ahmad Bakry, Dr. Mona Al Sane, Ms. Dina Ezzat, and Dr. Ameed Abdeulhamid of London.

My family support was immense, and I thank my mother, father, and brother Hesham, who focused their prayers towards asking God that this book come to reality. Thanks to all of you.

I also would like to offer a special thanks to my executive team: Ms. Enjy Mohammad, my secretary; Mr. Ahmad Hanafy, my office manager; Dr. El Hefnawy, my assistant in Cairo; Dr. Hayati, my assistant in Alexandria; and Dr. Shawkat, my senior assistant, who all provided a sincere effort to this work.

A special note of appreciation also goes to those who did the graphic work of this book: Ms. Nilly Ali and Mr. Khaled Eldawy.

Finally, I would like to thank every single person from the working team of Iowa State Press who contributed to the success of this book especially Mrs. Lynne Bishop, the project manager of this book.

RECONSTRUCTIVE AESTHETIC IMPLANT SURGERY

1
Introduction

Abd El Salam El Askary

ANCIENT COSMETICS

"The beauty has come" is what her name meant, and yet Nefertiti did not rely on her natural looks alone.[1] Her darkened eyebrows and boldly outlined eyes are as popular today as they were in the pharaonic times.

The art of cosmetic beautification has roots dating back to antiquity; famous pop star Billy Idol's distinctive hairdo (spikes) can be dated back to the end of the Iron Age (1000 B.C. to 50 B.C.), when Celts and Gauls used to wash their hair with limewater—a white, chalky substance—in an attempt to create striking white spikes of hair. Tattooing the whole body with blue pigments was a common practice in the late thirteenth century as depicted in the famous movie *Braveheart*.

The use of cosmetics in history was not restricted to the pharaohs' times; it can also be seen during the Paleolithic Age.[2] The curlers used by women today are actually an ancient beauty ritual followed by men and women alike. One of the earliest examples of hair curling is seen in Venus of Willendorf, a mummy belonging to the Paleolithic Age.[2]

Archeological evidence suggests that prehistoric people contrived their own techniques for preparing pigments for cosmetics. As many as seventeen different colors were reported to have been created from a few primary sources: lead, chalk, or gypsum (for white); charcoal (for black); and manganese ores (for shades of red, orange, and yellow). These pigments were blended with greasy substances to acquire the right consistency for painting on bodies.

For the ancient Egyptians, life was not as important as the afterlife, and their desire to look appealing extended beyond the grave. From the large amounts of perfumes and makeup found buried with the dead, we know that these were indispensable funerary gifts.[1]

So far, no one has ever found a sample of ancient Egyptian lipstick. However, the Louvre Museum in Paris gives us an indication that Nefertiti had perhaps attempted painting her lips. Surprisingly, both men and women of the upper classes used ground ants' eggs to paint their eyelids. The dye from the Henna plant was used to color hair and fingernails and to adorn the palms and soles of their feet. To freshen their breath they chewed on natron, a naturally occurring sodium carbonate.[3] Ancient chemists synthesized the black or gray makeup, referred to as *mesdemet* by the ancient Egyptians, that later acquired the name *kohl* from Arabs.[4]

Raw essences were brought from neighboring Mediterranean countries to be utilized for making perfumes, creams, and lotions, which were then exported. Scents constituted a large percentage of Egypt's exports at one time. Beauty inventions of the pharaohs spread so far that women belonging to the Roman Empire began to rely on cosmetics brought from Egypt and the other parts of the region.

Records have shown that the Sumerians, Babylonians, and Hebrews employed these compounds as much as the Egyptians for ceremonial, medicinal, and ornamental purposes. Locally, however, their use was most often confined to mummification rituals.

According to researchers, the apparent beauty of royal women in ancient times was essentially due to their ability to use natural resources to enhance their appearance.[4] They believed that makeup was only an adjuvant to one's own natural beauty.

Beautification and adornment are mutually inclusive terms that involve the use of cosmetics, clothing, jewelry, body piercing, tattooing, and so forth. They are fueled by a subconscious drive to look attractive and to feel good about ourselves. We also enjoy the attention we get from others when they notice our attractiveness,[5] which explains the contemporary high demand for cosmetics by all classes of society.

COSMETICS VERSUS AESTHETICS

The term *cosmetic* refers to substances and procedures that are used to enhance or correct defects in the appearance. Cosmetics are the preparations used to change the appearance or enhance the beauty of the face, skin, or hair. *Aesthetics,* on the other hand, signifies "natural beauty," a quality that comes from within. It can be defined as the science of beauty that is applied in nature and in art.

BEAUTY IN ART

Beauty is generally described as "a pleasurable psychological reaction to a visual stimulus," while the word *art* is derived from the Latin *ars,* meaning "skill."[6] For an artwork to be valued as good, it has to be satisfactory to the senses—what is referred to in the visual arts as "the relationships among colors, lines, and masses in space."[7]

People usually interpret beauty differently; each defining it according to his own conception. Prominent artistic figures have expressed their viewpoints about beauty in ways that are worth mentioning. In his *Vision of the Prophet,* Kalil Gibran manipulated magnificent pieces of poetry and prose to express his view of natural beauty: "Beauty is that which attracts your soul, and that which loves to give and not to receive."[8]

Dante also viewed art to as a natural imitation: "Art as far as it is able, follows nature, as a pupil imitates his master."

Leonardo da Vinci's famous Mona Lisa, the enigmatic woman whose identity remains a mystery to this day, reveals his perspective on beauty.[9] In the Mona Lisa, da Vinci finds real "natural" beauty. The mysterious smile on her face—which could be interpreted as either angel-like or quite devilish—was the secret of her everlasting beauty.[10]

Most artists have one thing in common: they use their talent to imitate reality—the real beauty they find in a certain thing, such as nature or the beauty of a face or soul. In this way, Peter Paul Rubens expressed his true feelings towards his beloved, Susanna Fourment, by imitating her beauty in "a portrait of my love."[10]

Art has always been instrumental in the imitation of beauty or nature. When Honoré de Balzac was once asked what art is, his reply was "nature concentrated." Thus, artists derive their inspiration from God's magnificent creation of nature and of us, and all artistic endeavors are compared to nature as the standard of excellence.

Like artists in their paintings, clinicians should attempt to maintain a balance of proportions in their work. Perfection cannot exist in isolation: each element of beauty must harmonize with all other related elements to create the whole. For example, a beautiful face cannot be called so unless all facial features are in harmony.

HARMONY IS THE KEY

The philosophy of beauty and beautification is so wide-ranging throughout history to the present time that it has attracted people of all kinds: artists, musicians, and even common man. It makes the clinician's task of attaining perfect aesthetics even more challenging. Like a musician composing the different elements that will orchestrate his music, a successful clinician integrates the treatment elements for a particular patient before executing the treatment plan (Fig. 1.1a,b).

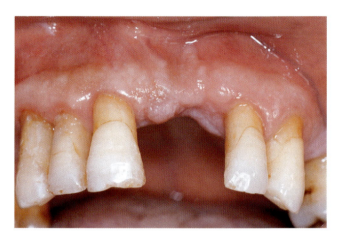

FIGURE 1.1a.   Preoperative view of a patient with a missing left central incisor.

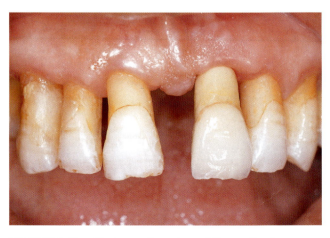

FIGURE 1.1b.   Postoperative view of the patient restored. Note the harmony between the implant-supported restoration and the remaining natural dentition.

Beauty in dentistry does not differ widely from the general art concepts that have been discussed earlier. Cosmetic dentistry as defined by Philips[11] is an elective procedure aimed at altering the existing natural or unnatural periodontium to a configuration perceived by the patient to enhance the appearance; on the other hand, aesthetic dentistry is a rehabilitative procedure that corrects a functional problem using techniques that will be least apparent in the remaining natural periodontium and/or associated tissues.[11] A successful aesthetic dental treatment should help the patient to regain his/her self-image, revive social skills, and experience professional success.

In evaluating an aesthetic treatment as successful, the clinician's visual judgment becomes very significant. That is, the success of an aesthetic procedure can be determined only when the eye moves along the object to be corrected and perceives its cohesion and harmony with all the other relevant aesthetic elements.[12] Any aesthetic restoration requires imaginative skills, superior clinical talents, and the comprehension of all facial relationships that will influence the treatment success. Logic and imagination are both necessary in analyzing the available elements that are required to ensure a harmonious aesthetic result.

There is a social dimension that complements the image of every person. Natural teeth are not mere physical structures with only a functional role to perform. They have social attributes as well, which are vital to one's self-image, social interaction, and physical attractiveness (Fig. 1.2). Restoring missing natural dentition, especially in the anterior area, has a complementary impact on the individual's personal and social countenance. Experience has proven that most patients not only perceive the functional improvements provided by prosthodontic rehabilitation, but also note remarkable improvements in their social and spiritual well-being as a result of the changes in their appearance.

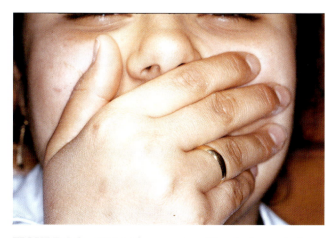

FIGURE 1.2. View of a woman with missing anterior dentition; she used to cover her mouth while laughing to hide her edentulous status.

Dental implants have proven to be a predictable method of restoring function in the oral cavity over the past thirty-five years.[13–16] The late 1980s and early 1990s witnessed the expansion of the use of dental implants to include treatment of partially edentulous patients with fixed, implant-supported restorations. These new clinical applications include the treatment of missing anterior single dentition, which has become a treatment option with documented success rates in excess of 90%.[17–20] As awareness of this treatment modality has improved, restoration of missing maxillary anterior single teeth with implant-supported restorations is quickly becoming the preferred treatment modality, despite the fact that it still remains one of the most aesthetically difficult and challenging of all implant restorations. Efforts by clinicians to improve the aesthetic dimension of dental implants and achieve restorations that exactly mimic the appearance of natural teeth have played a significant role in improving the awareness and popularity of dental implants.

Success in achieving an aesthetic implant-supported restoration that mimics the natural tooth appearance requires very meticulous treatment procedures. The process involves careful, detailed presurgical planning, optimal three-dimensional implant placement, meticulous soft tissue management, the use of predictable bone grafting techniques when required, and skillful use of various prosthetic components.

Many researchers have dedicated their efforts to improving and developing techniques that help achieve predictable, aesthetic results with dental implants. Some have laid out the fundamentals of presurgical planning,[21] and others[22,23] have set the guidelines for aesthetic implant positioning to achieve a natural-looking final restoration.

Soft tissue sculpture,[24] the use of connective tissue grafts[25] and free gingival grafts,[26] improvement of soft tissue contours,[27] the use of enhanced conservative new mucoperiosteal flap designs,[28] and methods to improve soft tissue topography at the time of second-stage surgery[29] were all invented to benefit the aesthetic outcome.

To achieve adequate height and width of the alveolar bone to obtain an optimal natural emergence profile, many techniques have been introduced.[30,31] Jovanovic[32] defined the term *aesthetic bone grafting* as the regeneration of the lost osseous structure to its original biological dimensions, not only to serve function but also to favor aesthetics.

Unlike natural dentition, restoring a single missing tooth with an implant-supported prosthesis can be a difficult task, never like restoring multiple missing teeth in the aesthetic zone.[33] In cases where only a single tooth is to be restored, the establishment of the peri-implant papillae and surrounding tissues is highly predictable,[34] whereas in the case of multiple implant placements the interimplant papilla is unpredictable. Some authors[35–38] have suggested soft tissue surgical interventions as a solution for this problem, while others[33,39] have utilized hard tissue reconstructive procedures. Tarnow[40] and Salama[41] have proposed helpful tools for predicting the inter- and peri-implant papillae with classifications that have assisted in the assessment of clinical papillary conditions. Misch[42] stated that aesthetic enhancement techniques are very often accomplished at the expense of sulcular health, as some of the clinical procedures can be invasive to peri-implant tissues. For example, creating deep soft tissue pockets around abutments can jeopardize the long-term survival of the implant and its surrounding structures.

Aesthetic implant dentistry should not be a separate discipline but rather an integral part of all other treatment modalities.[43] Function should complement aesthetics and vice versa: the final objective of aesthetic implant dentistry is a perfect prosthetic outcome that simulates the natural tooth appearance. Simple principles of design applied to anterior dental aesthetics that create harmony while maintaining natural beauty can turn an average restorative case into an ideal one. [44]

There is no right or wrong when it comes to an aesthetic restoration. It is the clinician's own responsibility to analyze the available treatment options and utilize the best possible working strategy that will provide a predictable long-term prognosis.

REFERENCES

1. Kunzig, Robert. Style of The Nile. Sept. 1999.
2. Faure, Elie. History of Art. Vol. 3, Renaissance Art. New York: Harper & Brothers Publishers, 1923.
3. Cosmetics. Microsoft(r) Encarta(r) Online Encyclopedia. 2000.
4. Breuer, M., ed. Cosmetic Science. 2 vols. 1978–80.
5. Boucher, Francois. 20,000 Years of Fashion: The History of Costume and Personal Adornment. New York: Harry N. Abrams, Inc., Publishers, 1965; Contini, Mila. Fashions from Ancient Egypt to the Present Day. London, 1965.
6. Encyclopedia of World Art, vol. 15. McGraw-Hill, 1959, 68.
7. Gombrich, Ernst. The Story of Art, 13th ed. London: Phaidon, 1978.
8. Gibran, Kahlil, ed., Vision of the Prophet. 1980.
9. Corson, Richard. Fashions in Makeup. London: Peter Owen, 1972.
10. Gunn, Fenja. The Artificial Face: A History of Cosmetics. London: Trinity Press, 1973.
11. Philips ED. The anatomy of a smile. Oral Health 1996(86): 7–9, 11–3.
12. Copper DF. Interrelationships between the visual art, science and technology. Leonardo 1980(13):29–33.
13. Brunski JB, et al. The influence of functional use of endosseous implants on the tissue-implant interface: Histological aspects. J Dent Res 1979 58(10): 1953–1969.
14. Adell R, Lekholm U, Rockler B. A 15 Year study of osseointegrated implants in the treatment of the edentulous jaw. Int J Oral Surg 1981(10): 387–416.
15. Engquist B, Bergendal T, Kallus T, et al. A retrospective multicenter evaluation of osseointegrated implants supporting overdentures. Int J Oral Maxillofac Implants 1988(3): 129–134.
16. Schnitman PA, Rubenstein JE, Whole PS, et al. Implants for partial edentulism. J Dent Educ 1988(52): 725–736.
17. Schmitt A and Zarb GA. The longitudinal clinical effectiveness of osseointegrated dental implants for single tooth replacement, Int J Prosthodont 1993(6): 187–202.
18. Engquist B, Nilson H, and Astrand P. Single tooth replacement by osseointegrated Brånemark implants: A retrospective study of 82 implants. Clin Oral Implant Res 1995(6): 238–245.
19. Anderson B, Odman P, Lidvall AM, et al. Single tooth restoration supported by osseointegrated implants: Results and experience from a prospective study after 2 to 3 years. Int J Oral Maxillofac Implants 1995(10): 702–711.
20. Ekfeldt A, Carlsson G, and Borgesson G. Clinical evaluation of single tooth restorations supported by osseointegrated implants. A retrospective study. Int J Oral Maxillofac Implants 1994(9): 179–183.
21. Jansen C, and Weisgold A. Presurgical treatment planning for the anterior single-tooth implant restoration. Compendium 1995(16): 746–762.
22. Spielman HP. Influence of the implant position on the aesthetics of the restoration. Pract Periodont Aesthet Dent 1996(8): 897–904.
23. Parel SM, and Sullivan, DY. Aesthetics and Osseointegration. Dallas, TX: Taylor Publishing Co., 1989, 11.
24. Bichacho N, and Landsberg CJ. A modified surgical prosthetic approach for an optimal single implant-supported crown, part I: The cervical contouring concept. Pract Periodont Aesthet Dent 1994(6): 35–41.
25. Khoury F, and Happe A. The palatal subepithelial connective tissue flap method for soft tissue management to cover maxillary defects: A clinical report. Int J Oral Maxillofac Implants 2000(15): 415–418.
26. Miller PD. Root coverage using a free soft tissue autograft following citric acid application. Part I: Technique. Int J Periodont Rest Dent 1982(2): 65–70.
27. Lazara RJ. Managing the soft tissue margin: The key to implant aesthetics. Pract Periodont Aesthet Dent 1993(5): 81–87.
28. Nemcovsky CE, Moses O, Artzi Z. Rotated palatal flap in immediate implant procedures. Clin Oral Implant Res 2000(11): 83–90.
29. Sharf DR, Tarnow DP. Modified roll technique for localized alveolar ridge augmentation. Int J Periodontics Restorative Dent 1992(12): 415–425.
30. Pikos M.A. Block autografts for localized ridge augmentation: Part II. The posterior mandible. Implant Dent 2000(9): 67–75.
31. Simion M, Trisi P, and Piatelli A. Vertical ridge augmentation using a membrane technique associated with osseointegrated implants. Int J Periodont Rest Dent 1994(14): 497–511.

32. Jovanovic SA. Bone rehabilitation to achieve optimal aesthetics. Pract Periodont Aesthet Dent 1997(9): 41–52.

33. El Askary AS. Interimplant papilla reconstruction by means of a titanium guide. Implant Dent 2000(9) 85–89.

34. Petrungaro PS. Smilanich MD, and Windmiller NW. The formation of proper interdental architecture for single tooth implants. Contemp Esthet Rest Pract 1999(3): 14–22.

35. Beagle JR. Surgical reconstruction of the interdental papilla: Case report. Int J Periodontics Restorative Dent 1992(12): 145–151.

36. Shapiro A. Regeneration of the interdental papillae using periodic curettage. Int J Periodontics Restorative Dent 1985(5): 27–33.

37. Jemt T. Regeneration of gingival papillae after single implant treatment, Int J Periodontics Restorative Dent 17(1997): 327–333.

38. Hurzeler MB, and Dietmar W. Peri-implant tissue management: Optimal timing for an aesthetic result. Pract Periodont Aesthet Dent 1996(8): 857–869.

39. Salama H, Salama MA, Garber D, and Adar P. Developing optimal peri-implant papilla within the esthetic zone: Guided soft tissue augmentation, J Esthet Dent 1995(7): 125–129.

40. Tarnow D, Magner A, and Fletcher P, The effect of the distance from the contact point to the crest of the bone on the presence or absence of the interproximal dental papilla. J Peridontol 1992(63): 995–996.

41. Salama H, Salama M, Garber D, and Adar P. The interproximal height of bone—a guide post to predictable esthetic strategies and soft tissue contours in anterior tooth replacement. Pract Periodont Aesthet Dent 1998(10): 1131–1141.

42. Misch EC. Single tooth implant. In Misch CE, ed. Contemporary Implant Dentistry. St. Louis: Mosby, 1999, 397–428.

43. Sorensen JA. Aesthetics at what cost? Pract Periodont Aesthet Dent 1997(9): 969–970.

44. Golub-Evans J. Unity and variety; essential ingredients of a smile design. Curr Opin Cosmet Dent 1994:1–5.

2
Presurgical Considerations

Abd El Salam El Askary

The quintessence of an optimal postsurgical aesthetic outcome is presurgical planning. One cannot imagine any difficult task being undertaken without thinking the whole procedure out very thoroughly prior to commencing on it. This crucial preplanning stage aims at fulfilling the patient's expectations at both the functional and aesthetic levels.

In general the patient goes to the dentist for help and guidance and for an honest opinion about what lies in his/her best interest. Therefore, the patient's expectations are in most cases what the clinician might seek to realize. However, the clinician must be prudent to be able to visualize what is feasible and realistic based on the existing clinical condition.

The dentist and his team make use of all available investigative tools to recommend and display all treatment options. It is the patient's right to be made aware not only of the possible use of dental implants but also of all other available treatment alternatives.

Imagination is a sign not only of creativity but also of farsightedness. The ability to envision the final treatment outcome before starting on it will help the dentist assess what is needed to restore the dentition and/or its supporting structures. If dental implants are to be considered, it is necessary that the final implant-supported restoration and related soft tissue margins should match and harmonize with the remaining natural counterparts. In this regard, selection of a clinical option that will ensure the best possible aesthetic result is of foremost importance.

Implant replacement therapy is not a traditional treatment option that can be taken lightly, or for granted, either in its course or in its final outcome. Successful long-term function of dental implant restorations requires a solid foundation of diagnosis, treatment planning, and case preparation. Bone and soft tissue volume, topography, and quality, differ, as do implant designs, surfaces, and surgical protocols. Each patient also has different requirements, desires, expectations, and a unique array of health concerns. Implant success thus requires a personalized approach, based on the functional, anatomical, aesthetic, and psychological needs of the implant candidate. Diagnosis and treatment planning are the starting point for achieving the treatment goals.

The patient must be notified of the benefits and potential complications of implant therapy. As mentioned earlier, the patient's expectations of the proposed treatment plan must be attended to conscientiously. It is the clinician's responsibility to inform the patient prior to treatment initiation about the extent of probable realization of his/her expectations.

Presurgical planning is not just limited to setting the groundwork for the patient. The treatment team must be well versed on everything related to the patient and the work required from every one of them. A well-prepared diagnostic study is one that will shed light on fundamental aspects of the oral cavity's anatomical structures and clinical condition. Areas of condition include type of occlusion; number, shape, and condition of the remaining dentition; and amount of interdental and interarch space available for replacement of teeth. The detection of any existing pathological lesion, parafunctional habits, or abnormal physiology should be underscored. This information is crucial in making critical decisions on the many aspects of treatment, each of which is important in its own right. These conditions mandate the position, size, type, and design of the future implants; the need for undertaking any grafting or bone augmentation procedures; the surgical approach; the positioning of the implant in the alveolar ridge; the selection of the prosthetic components; and the type of future restoration. Therefore, the diagnostic information obtained prior to treatment initiation can provide valuable insight into the appropriate sequence that is to be followed during the surgical and restorative phases of treatment.

A patient undergoing a comprehensive aesthetic reconstruction in the oral cavity has to be provided with a detailed description of the treatment procedures. The patient has his/her own crucial role in this whole treatment process. It is only fair that he/she know the extent of the required participation and what is expected of him/her during and after treatment. Another point of importance is the time frame and costs involved, which must also be presented and discussed at this time.

The patient must be informed of any possible discomfort, pain, or temporary compromise in function that he/she might experience, and a patient seeking implant replacement therapy requires reassurance to attain the patience and endurance demanded for investigating, preparing, and executing the selected treatment plan that will pay off at the end of the treatment. Consequently, it is only humane for the clinician to try to minimize the time of the actual treatment. The ideal presurgical planning can significantly reduce the time required for treatment, and subsequently minimizes unnecessary financial burdens and strains.

A clinician of these days may not depend only on visual and palpable examination of the visible oral vital structures; the underlying investing structures also must be thoroughly examined. Radiographic, modern diagnostic evaluation tools are thus reckoned as stepping-stones for the ensuing treatment. These are the necessary ingredients for any successful aesthetic project, and this pretreatment appraisal influences not only treatment modality selection but also treatment timing, sequence, and prognosis. Various available radiographic views can help assess the quantity, quality, and inclination of the residual alveolar ridge. Such related anatomical details as the nasal floor, maxillary sinus, and anterior mental looping may also be identified. Any pathology or bone disease related to the working site may be detected and dealt with before treatment commencement. Preoperative radiographs may be of assistance when reviewing with the patient the progress made during the course of the treatment and for comparison postoperatively. In the event of future medicolegal problems, radiographs are used as evidence of the patient situation at present and both pre- and postoperatively.

Besides radiographs, old photographs or slides the patient might provide are regarded as fairly important tools in constructing the treatment plan. The patient may yearn to duplicate what he or she previously looked like,

or may wish to hide some deformity or abnormality that he/she might used to have. Learning the patient's desires and expectations using old previous pictures as a reference can be very helpful in anterior oral rehabilitations.

Study casts are yet another useful tool in this stage of planning. They are made preoperatively from casting a preliminary impression. The type of occlusion and the available interarch space are the two major important benefits of study casts.

Therefore, it is imperative that the clinician seek to obtain the most information possible before starting the treatment. There are several means of acquiring this information. The first of these is similar to a background check, where the patient's medical and dental history is investigated.

MEDICAL EVALUATION

A complete medical and dental history provides insight into the patient's current state of health. It highlights contraindications or important areas of concern for dental implant therapy,[1,2] and it can also provide useful information on the potential success of implant treatment.[3,4,5] The following areas of medical risks[6] associated with dental implant placement can be evaluated through a detailed medical history. Surgical and anesthetic risks including cardiovascular, respiratory, and renal diseases are major concerns that should be first carefully evaluated through the medical history.[6] Because the human body is a precise interrelated mechanism, there are many medical conditions that negatively affect osseointegration, and they should be noted.[6] These conditions include blood dyscrasias (e.g., anemia, leukemia, bleeding/clotting disorders, etc.), severe endocrine systemic diseases (e.g., uncontrolled diabetes, hyperthyroidism, pituitary/adrenal disorders, etc.), severely compromised immune systems (e.g., AIDS), severe gastrointestinal diseases (e.g., hepatitis, malabsorption, etc.), and severe musculoskeletal diseases (e.g., osteoporosis, osteopetrosis, etc.).

Other conditions that may require consideration in decision making are musculoskeletal diseases (e.g., severe osteoarthritis) and neurologic disorders (e.g., stroke, palsy, mental retardation, etc.), which may render a patient incapable of maintaining adequate oral hygiene on a daily basis.[6]

Some situations or predicaments preclude the success of implant therapy because they compromise the body's health either generally or locally. Pregnancy, persistent oral infections, and malignancies are examples of such contraindicating situations for dental implant therapy.[7]

Relative contraindications to dental implant therapy, on the other hand, are conditions that are debilitating to the body's immune system. Although they do not directly pose a potential threat to dental implant survival, these contraindications would eventually be the cause of failure of implant acceptance within the host body. These relative contraindications include prolonged corticosteroid or immunosuppressive drug therapy, chemotherapy, collagen diseases, and a history of osteomyelitis or irradiation in the region of the proposed implant receptor site.[7] Patients are urged to reveal any ongoing medical treatment and/or any medications they are taking as well as any influencing habits. Smoking is increasingly cited in the literature as a risk factor in soft tissue healing,[8] periodontal health,[9,10] and implant therapy.[11–15]

Allergies are yet another source of concern. A thorough medical and dental history is important in identifying allergies that could dictate the use or avoidance of certain drugs or other substances in dental implant therapy. Due to its high passivity and biocompatibility, no allergies to titanium or titanium alloy have been reported in the dental literature.[16–18] However, allergies to denture resin[19] and such restorative base metals as chromium-cobalt,[16,19] nickel,[18–19] and palladium-copper-gold alloys[20] have appeared in research abstracts.

It is important to note that the literature suggests evaluating medically compromised implant candidates on a patient-by-patient basis, as compromised medical status alone is not necessarily indicative of implant failure.[20]

Physical conditions and symptoms are not the only aspects an oral surgeon should evaluate and assess. A patient's psychological ability to commit to long-term treatment and maintenance programs must be an integral part of the examination and selection process. During the consultation, the clinician should determine whether the patient is psychologically capable of making the necessary long-term commitment. For example, phobic or highly anxious individuals may have low pain thresholds and refuse to present for treatment follow-ups. On the other hand, patients whose dental complaints stem from somatization disorders will probably not be satisfied with the results of implant therapy.[21]

It is unfortunate that not every person may be considered mentally, psychologically, physically, and emotionally sound. As a result, some cases may contraindicate for dental implant therapy. Persons afflicted with acute psychiatric or psychological disorders are one such example.[6] These disorders may be subdivided into (a) inability to understand information, follow instructions, or make reasonable decisions (e.g., psychotic syndromes, severe neurotic conditions, or character disorders, etc.); (b) impaired memory or motor coordination necessary for routine oral hygiene (e.g., cerebral lesion syndromes, pre-

senile dementia, etc.); and (c) chronic, severe alcohol or drug addiction (because of a high propensity for poor motivation, inadequate nutrition, and lack of compliance with oral hygiene regimen).[22] As always, it is best to select candidates whose level of understanding and cooperation is superior, for that guarantees a successful end result.

Registering information and taking notes on past history is only one aspect of the presurgical stage of implant therapy. A thorough physical examination prior to implant placement is imperative in order to assess the patient's present health status and detect early signs of an undiagnosed disease.[22] Recording the patient's vital signs (pulse, blood pressure, respiratory rate, and temperature) can be important in assessing the patient's present overall health. Other medical tests and/or consultation with the patient's physician may be necessary when compromised medical conditions exist.

A comprehensive hard and soft tissue examination should be performed in order to rule out undiagnosed malignancies or dysplastic oral, head, and neck lesions.[22] Inspection and bidigital palpation of the lips, buccal mucosa, hard and soft palates, the oral pharynx and the submental, submandibular, and cervical lymph nodes should be made to assess the presence of any masses.[22] By gently grasping and lifting the tongue forward, upward and laterally, the floor of the mouth and the tongue can also be examined.[22]

The salivary glands and ducts must be inspected for unobstructed asymptomatic salivary flow that might cause lack of lubrication to any oral prosthesis and may mandate a change in the proposed prosthodontic plan.

STUDY CAST

The study cast is considered to be a valuable diagnostic tool that assists in developing and executing the treatment plan (Fig. 2.1).[23] This is primarily due to the fact that the patient can only be examined for a limited time per visit. The study cast provides an almost exact replica of the oral conditions prevailing at the time the impression is made. Transferring the patient's intraoral condition to a dental cast is a vital prerequisite to presurgical planning; it enables the clinician to study and comprehend the treatment elements needed to satisfy all the aesthetic and functional demands in subsequent treatment phases.[24] The master study cast may be duplicated two or three times for various clinical applications. One duplicate may be used in fabricating the surgical template, another in constructing a provisional restoration for the patient, and another may be retained and preserved as a record for any future demand.

The uses of study casts are numerous, especially since they provide information that is measurable and verifi-

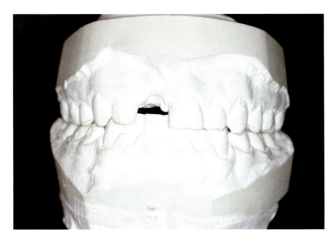

FIGURE 2.1. Study casts mounted on a simple hinge articulator showing a missing maxillary right central incisor.

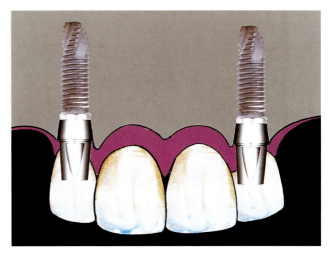

FIGURE 2.2. An illustration showing the use of a reduced number of implants to enable enhanced peri-implant soft tissue architecture.

able. They are helpful in determining the interarch space and sulcus depth. These measurements are necessary in order to calculate the future crown-implant ratio, the type of implant used, the type of the final abutment, and the extent of the final restoration.[27]

Study casts can also lend a hand in determining the number and size of implants to be used in supporting a given prosthesis. In areas where function is of prime importance, as in replacing missing posterior dentition, a maximum number of implants should be used to provide a larger surface area for support. This procedure is recommended as a safety factor so that the implants can withstand the magnified stresses at these particular areas, ensuring a better prognosis. Whereas, in areas where aesthetics are desirable and biting forces are at a minimum, it is the personal experience of the author that sometimes reducing the number of implants used (without compromising the function) can strikingly improve the aesthetic outcome by enhancing peri-implant soft tissue architecture. The availability of a pontic space between the implants allows the clinician to perform pontic development techniques, resulting in a papillary-like architecture that simulates natural appearance (Figs 2.2, 2.3a–c).[25,26] When a reduced number of implants is used to execute pontic development techniques, longer and surface-enhanced implants should be used to provide a reasonable support for the long-term success of the implant-supported prosthesis.

Study casts can occasionally give a valuable indication of the nature of available osseous support. They can be useful in assessing the amount of bone required from a proposed grafting procedure to contribute to the long-term serviceability and improved aesthetics of the dental implants. In conjunction with the available radiographic

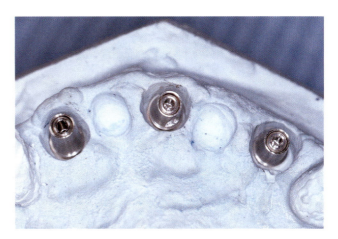

FIGURE 2.3a. A master cast showing the use of three implants to restore five missing anterior teeth; note the sculpture of the pontic area on the model.

views, study casts aid in the accurate selection of implant size by determining the bone width at a given section of the alveolar ridge using a technique called ridge mapping.[28,29] This involves inserting a thin needle or a tissue gauge into the soft tissue investing the alveolar ridge following a vertical line drawn in the middle of the edentulous area or at the area of intrest. The measurement is repeated at two or three locations along the vertical line both facially and lingually. The collected depth readings are then transferred onto the corresponding locations on the sectioned study cast at the same vertical line. These readings furnish the thickness of the soft tissue. Additionally, the underlying bone width can be calculated by subtraction (Figs 2.4a–d). This technique can be used to reduce the cost of the treatment (by eliminating the fees

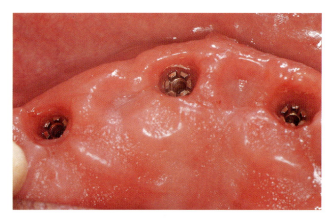

FIGURE 2.3b. Final clinical result after pontic development technique. Note the formed papillary-like architecture.

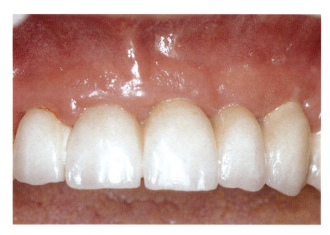

FIGURE 2.3c. Final restoration cemented in place restoring the natural emergence and papillary architecture.

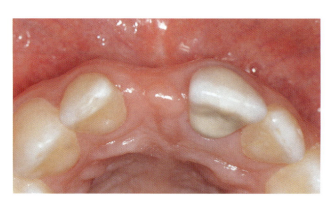

FIGURE 2.4a. Incisal view of a missing right central incisor showing labial bone defect due to postextraction resorption.

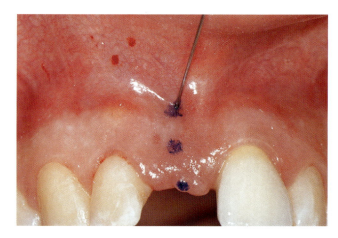

FIGURE 2.4b. Three pin markings labially and three pin markings palatally are made. A needle punching the soft tissue at the markings place to record the soft tissue depth is shown.

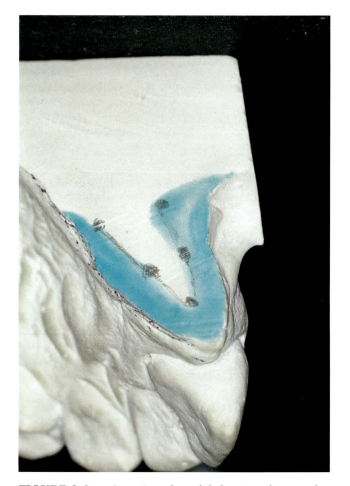

FIGURE 2.4c. A sectioned model showing the actual thickness of bone after tracing the collected data; the blue color represents the soft tissue thickness.

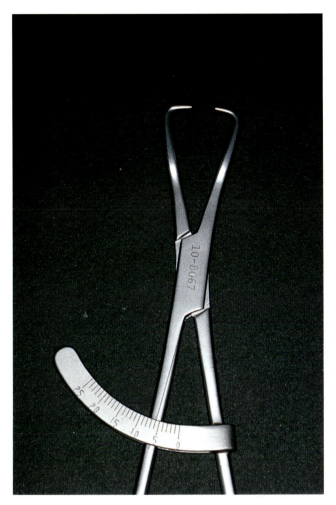

FIGURE 2.4d. A tissue gauge caliper can be used instead of the needle puncture to measure soft tissue depth.

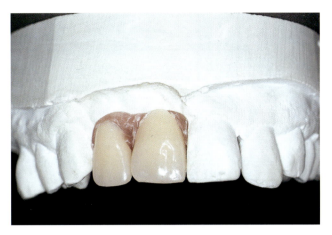

FIGURE 2.5. A wax-up of two missing anterior teeth on the study model.

for CT scans) and to eliminate the exposure to radiation (to satisfy some patients' preferences).

The study cast is not limited in its use to obtaining information and taking measurements; after studying the available edentulous space and determining the number of implants required, a wax-up (Fig. 2.5) is subsequently fabricated to replace the missing natural dentition, and reestablish the missing biological contours. In effect, the wax-up on the study cast is very much like a dress rehearsal. It is then shown to the patient so he/she can evaluate it personally and directly on the study cast. This makes the whole treatment process more tangible for the patient. However, evaluation of the wax-up is usually complicated for the patient because it is difficult for him/her to imagine and visualize him-/herself with a new prosthesis from simply observing a wax-up.[30] Examples of attempts made to enhance the realistic appearance of the wax-up for the patient include placing a pink matrix

around the teeth, by painting, or using tooth-colored and pink base plate wax to simulate gingival appearance.[31] Sometimes adding a lip impression to the pink matrix on the study cast will provide a three-dimensional vision for the patient.[32] After the patient approves the wax-up, the locations of the future implants are marked on the cast. A surgical template constructed on the study cast according to the markings of these locations will aid in transferring the planned first stage of surgery onto the surgical site.

In conclusion, the study cast is the main diagnostic tool in the presurgical phase, as it aids in evaluating the edentulous space in relation to the number, location, and/or size of the missing dentition. It also helps in analyzing the biomechanical forces exerted, detecting the type of occlusion, and determining the prosthetic components to be used in the future. Other nondiagnostic functions include fabrication of the surgical template as well as any provisional prostheses. Additionally, the study cast may be used as a reference guide for comparison between the different stages of the treatment, thus evaluating the treatment progress. If medicolegal problems should arise, the study cast may be considered and used as a material of evidence.

RADIOGRAPHIC ASSESSMENT

Implant positioning in the alveolar ridge is dependent on the location and morphology of the potential osseous receptor site and its contiguous structures. Because the contour and thickness of the oral mucosa can mask the actual dimensions of the underlying osseous structure, a thorough radiographic examination is essential for diagnosis and treatment. This examination is to make note of what is and is not radiographically present, with any deviation from normality duly recorded.[33]

Radiographic assessment is a significant tool in evaluating the quantity and the quality of the alveolar bone, locating any anatomical landmarks, and/or detecting pathological lesions. It helps the clinician to visualize and judge the likelihood of executing the proposed treatment plan. In addition to determining bone dimensions accurately,[34] the available technical advancements in radiography have helped improve case design and treatment planning, thus conferring upon clinical results a measure of predictability.[35] This, in turn, has helped the dental team select the proper candidate for implant therapy; implant size and design; surface texture and angulation; and the surgical technique to be utilized for implant placement.

There are numerous radiological techniques and views available, and each has its own merits and drawbacks. The clinician should be able to select the most suitable method for each patient particularly. Sophisticated radiography, as digital computed scans, is not mandatory for every single alveolar ridge evaluation. However, some patients require sophisticated radiographic investigations for assurance of attaining a successful treatment plan.

Periapical and panoramic views are examples of two very commonly used views in dental treatment. They offer only a two-dimensional image, where bone height and density may be gauged.[35] These views can also be helpful in evaluating the condition of the periodontium or pulp. They are also used to assess the location of the roots relative to the neighboring anatomical structures and/or a particular future implant receptor site. Acquiring periapical and panoramic x-ray views is cost effective, as the radiographic devices can be readily available in the dental office, are easy to use, and involve minimal additional expense for the patient.

The periapical view has a unique advantage over other types and views of x rays. It is the only available method for routine monitoring of crestal bone levels around previously restored dental implants. It can also be a valuable reference that the clinician can resort to at the time of surgery to determine the depth of drilling (Fig. 2.6).

Conversely, periapical radiography has some inherent shortcomings. These inadequacies are represented in a slight magnification of images that is not consistent and that varies according to the technique used. Consequently, an image in a periapical film doesn't represent the actual size of an object. Another disadvantage is the small size of the film, which restricts the viewed area, thus limiting its clinical applications. Periapical radiographs, however, are considered valuable in the treatment planning for single tooth implants.

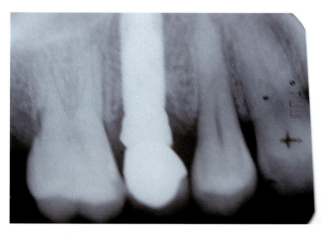

FIGURE 2.6. Periapical radiographic view.

Modern periapical digital radiographs have reduced 90% of the radiation exposure. They have eliminated the need for films and subsequent film processing. The regular film is replaced with a sensor that is connected to a computer, where the image can be viewed instantaneously.[36] The radiation reduction has benefited both the clinician and the patient, where digitalization has allowed for taking several views in a shorter time without fear of radiation hazard. It is thought to be cost effective in comparison with the regular radiographic views.

Occlusal views have very limited applications because of superimposition of anatomical structures, changes in the x-ray tube angulation that can lead to distortion in most of the images, and difficulties encountered in accessing the posterior regions of the oral cavity (Fig. 2.7).[37]

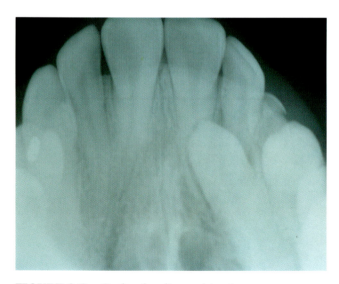

FIGURE 2.7. Occlusal radiographic view.

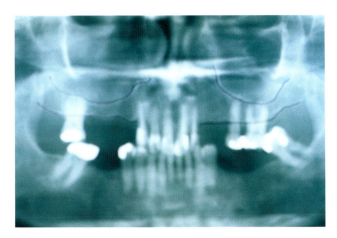

FIGURE 2.8. Panoramic view showing all the dentition and tracing of the maxillary sinus floor level with some anatomical landmarks (note the image magnification).

Panoramic radiography (Fig. 2.8) is believed to be the standard technique for radiographic examination in the treatment planning for patients receiving dental implants.[38,39] It shows the hard and soft tissue anatomy and the related structures of the maxilla and mandible in a single film. However, although it is considered the most popular two-dimensional view in oral implantology treatment, it has its own shortfalls: it fails to show the width of the object. Panoramic views also have lower resolution (especially in the anterior zone) than intraoral radiographs. Moreover, when these radiographs are magnified to 15–22%, it is difficult to calculate the exact bone height, or mesiodistal distance, without performing a mathematical calculation to eliminate the magnification factor. In spite of its disadvantages, however, panoramic radiography will remain the radiographic examination tool of choice in dental implant treatments because of its simplicity and affordability.

Periapical and panoramic views are not the only views that are applicable in dental implantology. Lateral cephalometric radiographs are usually used in order to focus on the anterior maxilla and mandible. Here, the trajectory and angulation of the residual alveolar ridge are required. Therefore, cephalographs provide information regarding the angulation of the implants to be placed. They are, however, limited in their application in dental implantology to completely edentulous patients.

Dental implants in general have benefited from computed dental radiography. Computerized tomography (CT), specifically, offers several advantages. It produces sharp images, eliminates the need for film processing, uti-

lizes a lower dose of radiation, presents precise measurements directly without magnification, and provides a digital image that can be stored on the computer for future comparisons.[37]

Computerized tomography (CT) is based on a software program that constructs a three-dimensional model. It creates clear tomographic sections for the alveolar bone, and differentiates between soft and hard tissues clearly as never before. It reformats the image data to create a tangential and cross-sectional tomographic image of the future implant site; it also verifies the bone quality precisely. This three-dimensional model is computed using several radiographic views from specific angles (Fig. 2.9a–e).[38] Because of its ability to provide a complete three-dimensional image, CT provides a highly sophisticated format for precisely defining jaw structure and locating critical anatomical structures.[23,39–42]

Dentascan (MPDI, Torrance, California) is considered to be one of the most modern applications of computerized tomography (CT) in implant dentistry. It generates a referenced cross-sectional and tangential panoramic image of the alveolar bone along with three-dimensional images of the arch. It consists of a software modification of the CT data to produce images specifically helpful for preoperative assessment of the alveolar bone before implant placement. It provides serial slices through the alveolar ridge at specific intervals. The surgeon is then able to visualize the alveolar bone in a three-dimensional image and measure the size of the ridge directly from the scan. This method has its limitations in terms of high cost, critical head tilting position of the patient, requiring a compensation for magnification, and the increased time needed for generation of the images.[43]

Magnetic resonance imaging may be used to appraise the existing alveolar bone, especially for use with dental implants. It is a useful scanning method that may be utilized in areas where CT software programs are not available, or for patients who don't desire or cannot be exposed to further radiation.[44]

To date, digital subtraction radiography (DSR) is the most versatile and sensitive method for measuring bone loss. It can detect both bone height and changes in bone mass surrounding dental implants. DSR addresses the limitations in detecting postoperative changes that are present in other radiographic modalities. By eliminating information that has not changed, DSR allows the clinician's eye to focus on actual changes that have occurred between the recordings of two images.[35,37] This feature makes comparison easier, and any uncertainties about the procedure's success can be laid to rest.

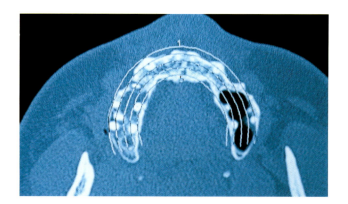

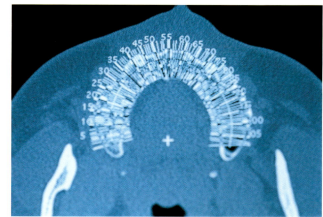

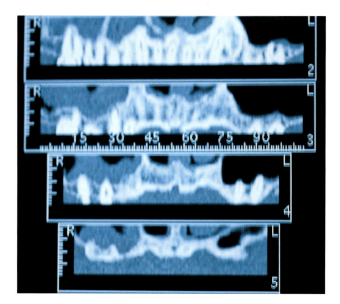

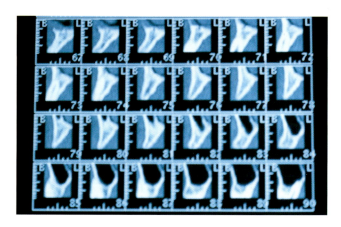

FIGURE 2.9a,b,c,d.   Four different views of a computerized tomography (CT) of the maxilla.

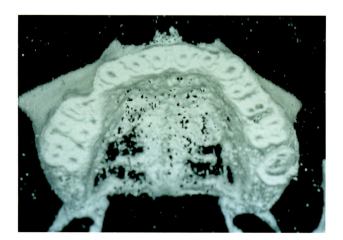

FIGURE 2.9e.   Three-dimensional simulation of the premaxilla from a CT.

Selection of the most suitable radiographic view requires rational decision and sound judgment. Sophis-
ticated and expensive radiographic procedures may sometimes not be helpful in detecting the various parameters needed to make a precise diagnosis, and the regular readily available radiographic techniques may be sufficient.

TREATMENT OPTIONS

Making sensible decisions is one of the most important daily activities of any clinician's practice. Currently obtainable data, statistical analysis methods, and technological advancements give the practitioner the facility to select a specific treatment path in a more thorough and predictable manner than ever before. When treating a partially or completely edentulous patient with dental implants, the primary target of the treatment should be determined: functional, aesthetic, or both. When aesthetics is a priority in the treatment plan, the patient should be actively involved in the details of the treatment plan, so as to accurately ascertain his/her aesthetic expectations.[45] It is crucial to conceive and comprehend what is in the patient's best interest prior to any aesthetic reconstructive methods being undertaken, in order to avoid any future medicolegal problems. Many disappointments may occur when a final prosthetic outcome does not satisfy the patient's wishes or meet his/her expectations. The reason may be due to poor clinician-patient communication, a misunderstanding of the patient's demands, and/or the dentist's inability to fulfill them.

All the available treatment options should be painstakingly explained to the patient prior to embarking on any clinical treatment procedures. The patient's gender, physical appearance, age, personality, cultural and ethnic background, profession, lifestyle requirements, and financial capability are all factors that will eventually influence the selection of a suitable treatment modality.[46]

There are various methods for restoring lost anterior teeth; these encompass conventional bridges, resin-bonded bridges, implant-supported restorations, removable partial dentures, or a combination of all of these various options.

Conventional Fixed Bridges

Fixed bridges have been for a long time the most ideal treatment modality for restoring natural dentition. They represented the school of thought in which aesthetics was of prime importance, even if the structure of the remaining natural teeth was compromised.

Conventional bridges have exhibited clinically proven high success rates with their excellent aesthetics and long-term functional serviceability.[47] However, in spite of their outstanding clinical performance, there is a significant variation in their success rates as documented in the literature, ranging from 97 to 80%.[48,49] These variations are probably due to differences in clinical performance, precision of the bridge fabrication, and the type of the metal alloy used.

The main reason for failure of conventional bridges is attributed to endodontic failure of the abutment teeth after an unknown period of time.[50] The extensive destruction of the abutment teeth through tooth preparation for conventional bridges is now considered to be a clinical drawback, especially when the teeth are sound. The immense loss of tooth structure during tooth preparation can be the actual reason for unsatisfactory results with this treatment option.

With the evolution of dental implants, preservation of natural teeth that would normally be used to serve as abutments for a fixed bridge has been emphasized. In other words, dental implants have paved the way for a shift in thought towards preservation of the remaining

natural teeth: dental implants are used to replace the missing tooth/teeth without resorting to including neighboring abutment teeth that are in a relatively good condition.

Using general standards that exist in the literature, the average lifetime of a fixed bridge is 8.3–10.3 years.[51,52] This might raise the question of how many restorations a young patient might require over a lifetime. Alternatively, if the teeth adjacent to an edentulous space have either severe attrition or a gross restoration, dental implants may not be a feasible treatment option. In this case, it would be better to consider protecting and splinting these compromised teeth within a bridge framework. Thus, the condition of the remaining dentition, the number of remaining dentition, parafunctional habits, type of occlusion, and leverage are all determinant factors that assist selection of this treatment modality.

Adhesive Bridges

An alternative treatment option that has been suggested in conserving and restoring missing dentition in the aesthetic zone is adhesive bridges. They eliminate the need for substantial destruction of natural abutments. Adhesive bridges were originally introduced by Rochette to be used as periodontal splints.[53] However, adhesive bridges present a treatment option that is different from conventional bridges. Adhesive bridges require greater clinical skills than do conventional bridges, and another point worth mentioning is the possibility of recurrent dental caries occurring around the bridge margins and line angles. De-bonding of adhesive bridges, which leads to loosening of the bridge, tends to occur at a frequency rate as high as 25–31%.[54,55] De-bonding tendency is considered the major complication of this type of bridge, which limits its regular daily use. Resin-bonded restorations have shown a wide range of clinical results as cited in the literature, from a failure rate of 54% in eleven months (when used in the absence of mechanical retentive methods) to a success rate of 92.9% in 127 cases (with a mean longevity of five years), as reported by Barrack.[56,57]

Resin-bonded bridges can only be suggested to a patient who is seeking a temporary, inexpensive aesthetic solution for a particular period of time. The specific nature of this treatment option should be explicitly explained to the patient.

Dental Implants

Unlike the previous alternatives, dental implants as a predictable treatment option have been investigated exhaustively over the past few years under controlled parameters, especially in completely edentulous patients.[58–60] Since the late eighties, continuous research and sophisticated statistical analysis have shown dental implants to be a predictable treatment option for dental restoration in totally and partially edentulous patients.[58]

The scope of dental implants later expanded to include the treatment of missing single teeth; this treatment has shown consistent success rates ranging from 91 to 97.4% over a 3–6 year period.[59,60] However, a few complications were encountered with this treatment modality; screw loosening has been reported most often as an uninvited event associated with single-tooth implant-supported restorations.[61] This drawback has been overcome to a great extent by the introduction of new implant-abutment connections that provide greater surface areas, stability against lateral displacement, and a predictable retention.

Implant dentistry has dramatically changed the conventional routine of restorative dentistry. It has inspired many clinicians who, in turn, have contributed to improving the clinical aesthetic outcome of this treatment modality. New soft and hard tissue augmentation procedures were developed to optimize the long-term aesthetic outcome of dental implants.[62] In partially edentulous patients, dental implants offer the advantage of eliminating the necessity of natural abutment preparation. They are considered to be the best tooth replacement alternative for both young and old patients because they preserve the structural integrity of the natural dentition. If the dental implant treatment should fail at any time, other treatment options would still be available as a next line of treatment, which makes this treatment modality unique in its kind. Moreover, retrospective and prospective studies have reported that dental implants have a positive effect on the recipient's well-being and quality of life, which has added a new social dimension to this treatment modality.[63]

Removable Partial Dentures

Removable partial dentures have been a treatment of choice when there are multiple missing teeth that may be dispersed throughout the dental arch and are not necessarily next to each other. This treatment option is also indicated when the remaining teeth are mobile and future extractions are expected. In addition, when patient resources are limited and the cost of treatment is a determining factor, the relative inexpensiveness of removable partial dentures becomes a good incentive for choosing this line of treatment.

However, as with other treatment options, partial dentures are not exempt from drawbacks. The possible occurrence of periodontal disease and natural tooth decay adjacent to the abutment teeth is one of the major disadvantages. Resorption of the alveolar ridge due to pressure from the fitting surface is another.[64–66] In addi-

tion, certain parts of the denture framework or acrylic resin can sometimes become visible while talking or smiling, which may not be aesthetically pleasing and thus may negatively contribute to the social dimension.[67] The aesthetic and functional outcome of fixed partial dentures, that is, conventional bridges, is regarded as being usually superior to that of a removable partial denture.[68]

In conclusion, making a removable partial denture is a feasible solution for patients who are unable to afford other treatment alternatives due to financial limitations or for whom other treatment modalities are contraindicated. It is also convenient for those who prefer not to undergo sophisticated treatment procedures that might involve soft and hard tissue grafting.

Points of Consideration

Prior to the final selection of the course of treatment to be undertaken, the patient must be made aware of the approximate total cost and time for the treatment involved. There are several steps required not only to insert an implant and its prosthetic components, but also to construct the overlying restoration and maintain the implant and its related components. The patient must have an active role in selecting a specific treatment plan from among several proposed ones; this role comes after thorough explanation of the pros and cons of each procedure proposed; this procedure splits the responsibility for treatment choice morally between the patient and the clinician.

An anterior implant-supported prosthesis invariably requires the clinician to spend more time, effort, and skill than replacements in the posterior zone. Sometimes additional corrective peri-implant soft tissue surgeries in the aesthetic zone are necessary; these consequently increase the overall cost of single anterior implant-supported restorations up to one-third of the total cost, and the time required for treatment completion is eventually doubled. Therefore, to avoid any disappointments or misunderstandings between the patient and the clinician, the approximate time and cost required for each treatment option should be a distinctive part of the doctor-patient preoperative communication that is confirmed with a signed consent by the patient.

It is also possible that the dentist may be biased towards a particular treatment plan, rather than following an objective approach.[69] This can happen when a clinician prefers certain procedures or is capable of performing some procedures better than others. Although this is not a recommended attitude, it is the clinician who is, at the end, responsible for the treatment choice and its results. Therefore, the clinician is urged to select a reasonable treatment option that both suits the patient's best interest and is compatible with the clinician's skills. This means catering to each patient's needs on an individual basis. Trustful dentist-patient communication remains critical and should be maintained throughout the course of treatment on both sides.

Patients seeking aesthetic treatment should be encouraged to understand and evaluate the entire scope of the clinical task to be carried out. When patients fully comprehend the extent of the work entailed, they will be able to appreciate it and convey a good impression to their personal contacts. In conclusion, the patient's positive attitude and greater willingness to cooperate during the treatment will surely lead to a better working environment for the dental team.

PROVISIONALIZATION PLANNING

As the word *provisional* suggests, provisionalization involves something that is used temporarily, to serve for a short period of time, until the permanent service is rendered. In this regard, its application to dental treatment is no exception. A critical stage in tooth replacement in the aesthetic zone is in the interim between implant insertion and surgical uncovering at the second-stage surgery. At this time, a provisional prosthesis may be used to temporarily restore the missing dentition and to maintain the social appearance of the patient. In fact, many patients, especially those who are "aesthetically conscious," ask a common question: Will I stay without teeth during the treatment? Although these patients may have been edentulous for years, their question can be explained as a turning point in their lives and a starting point for a new social and aesthetic era to be fulfilled. The provisional prostheses should be designed to sustain or improve the quality of life for patients undergoing implant therapy.[70]

A provisional prosthesis can be a valuable aid in determining the final tooth position, exact tooth shade, and occlusal scheme of the definitive prosthesis. Moreover, it can reveal any additional requirements for improved aesthetics and patient comfort.[70] The type of provisional prosthesis should be determined during the presurgical planning phase by the dental team.[70] A provisional restoration can be necessary to guide healing of the soft tissues around dental implants to develop the emergence profile until it reaches the original anatomical dimensions; this can minimize the need for further soft tissue manipulation.[71] The main advantage of the interim prosthesis is that it acts as a reference in designing the final prosthesis.[72]

When considering a provisional prosthesis for a patient who will receive an implant-supported restoration, the available options are removable partial denture, resin-bonded bridge, or temporary implants.

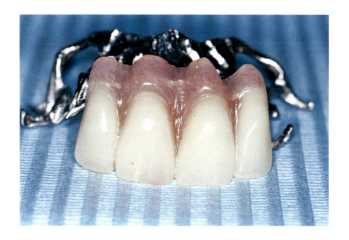

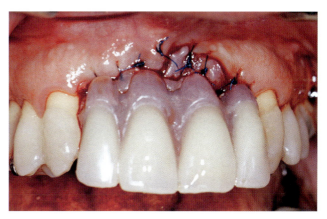

FIGURE 2.10a,b. Removable partial denture is used to provisionally restore four missing anterior teeth during the grafting and implant integration period.

Removable partial dentures can be indicated when there are adjacent or scattered multiple missing teeth (Fig. 2.10a,b). Being removable can be an advantage by itself: this facility is important during surgical intervention, as the partial dentures can be removed and then replaced once the procedure has been completed without any clinical complexity. Removable dentures also act as a stimulus for bone remodeling around dental implants in totally edentulous patients and can be used to confirm osseointegration before the final prosthesis is constructed.[73] This type of provisional solution provides an inexpensive provisional modality that must be taken into account based on the patient's financial status. The patient may feel psychologically improved with the edentulous area temporarily restored and other related facial structures being supported. However, the patient should be reminded that the prosthesis is only a temporary alternative for the missing space.

Removable partial dentures can be limiting in their function, especially during speaking or chewing, due to instability. Furthermore, some precautions need to be observed when removable partial dentures are used as a provisional modality for totally or partially edentulous patients; the appliance must be relieved from its fitting surface on top of the implant heads to avoid any biting load being exerted on the implants during the healing period. In addition, the material lining of the denture tends to dry out or become stiff over a period of use. This can be handled by changing the lining material at monthly intervals to maintain the elasticity of the fitting surface of the denture.

A resin-bonded bridge, on the contrary, does not exert any pressure on the implant area. It is better tolerated by the patient and may be more reassuring than a removable partial denture because of the improved aesthetic results, stability and fixation. However, a resin-bonded bridge can be a deterrent when multiple reentries to the surgical site are required (Fig 2.11a–c).

Temporary implants are bringing in a new era for provisionalization. They are commercially available from several companies and have solved many clinical prob-

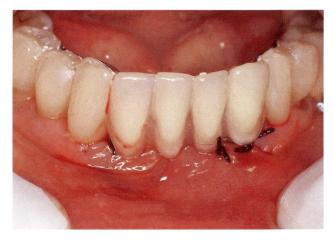

FIGURE 2.11c. Provisional resin-bonded bridge cemented in place after implant placement, thus restoring the patient aesthetics and function.

lems, especially for totally edentulous patients. They are self-tapping screws that have a diameter ranging between 1.8 and 2.8 mm and come in an assortment of various lengths. They are fabricated from either grade one commercially pure titanium or tritium alloy. These implants are inserted through a one-stage drilling procedure (only a pilot drill) with minimal surgical intervention. They should be placed at least 1 mm from the site of the permanent implants to avoid interrupting osseointegration around the implant-bone interface. They can be easily removed by reversed torque or by using a small diameter trephine drill after completion of the healing period for the permanent implants. They can be a reliable treatment alternative for patients who refuse to wear a removable prosthesis.[74] Temporary implants exhibit several advantages, including the possibility of providing immediate function after implant placement, uneventful soft tissue healing on top of the permanent implants, and restoration of phonetics and aesthetics.[75]

Improper placement of transitional implants can cause damage to a previously reconstructed alveolar ridge or jeopardize osseointegration around permanent implants. Another drawback is the difficulty of using these implants in the restoration of a single missing tooth due to lack of space (Fig. 2.12a,b). Transitional implants can be an ideal treatment option when more than two implants are to be inserted. This can be accomplished by placing a temporary implant positioned between the permanent fixtures or in a lingual position if the width of the alveolar bone allows.

The previously mentioned interim restorations are considered as a major part of the whole definitive treatment plan for patients receiving dental implants. Patients seeking aesthetic treatment should be encouraged to understand the entire scope of the clinical task to be car-

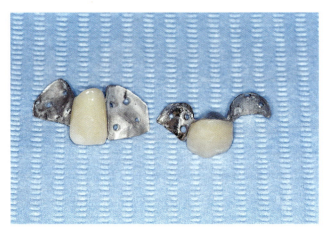

FIGURE 2.11a. Resin-bonded bridge.

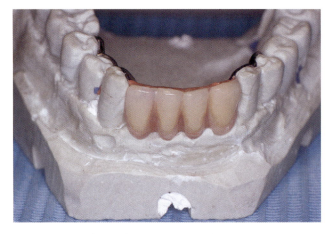

FIGURE 2.11b. A long-span resin-bonded bridge on a study cast.

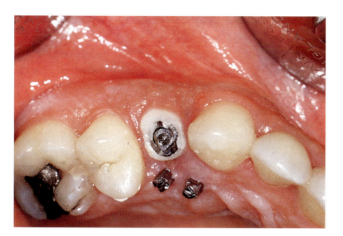

FIGURE 2.12a. Two transitional implants used to support a provisional restoration along with the temporary abutment.

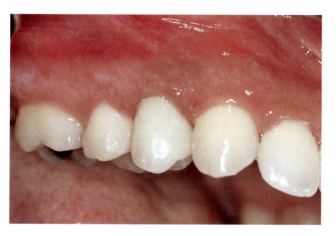

FIGURE 2.12b. The provisional restoration in place; note that it has its support mainly on the two transitional implants and partially on the temporary abutment.

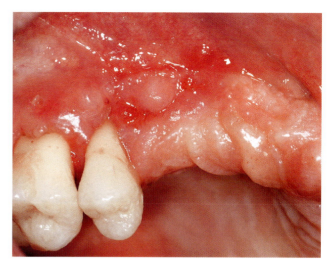

FIGURE 2.13a. An edentulous area showing soft tissue defects at the future implant sites that mandates correction before implant placement.

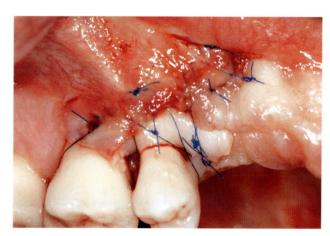

FIGURE 2.13b. A subepithelial soft tissue graft combined with the coronally repositioned flap is performed in order to improve the soft tissue status.

ried out. When patients fully comprehend the extent of work entailed, they will be able to appreciate it and accept the difficulties that might occur during the period of the treatment.

SOFT TISSUE QUALITY AND QUANTITY

Aesthetics in the anterior region relies heavily on healthy keratinized gingival tissue; this fact applies to both natural dentition and implant-supported restorations.[76] Gingival components that contribute to an aesthetically pleasing implant-supported restoration are the marginal radicular form, the interdental tissues, and the color and texture of healthy keratinized tissues (Fig 2.13a–c).[77]

Meticulous assessment of the soft tissue status related to the future implant site should be established during the clinical examination at the presurgical stage. The healthy soft tissue profile plays a critical role not only in establishing optimal aesthetics, but also in facilitating long-term maintenance of implant-supported restorations.[78] Some authors have shown conclusive results concerning the relationship between the condition of soft tissue and the implant survival; they concluded that neither the absence of inflamed soft tissue nor a specific amount of keratinized mucosa is required to ensure a successful osseointegration.[79,80] On the contrary, some authors have confirmed that the absence of a keratinized mucosa might jeopardize implant survival.[81,82] In addition, some authors have stated that a minimum of 2 mm of keratinized tissue

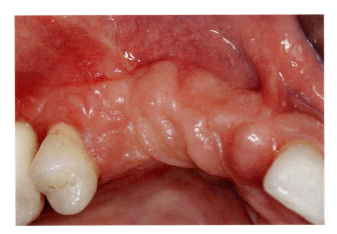

FIGURE 2.13c. The final soft tissue condition after clinical intervention; note the continuity of the keratinized band.

Two different distinctive periodontal patterns are present in the human oral cavity: the thin scalloped biotype and the thick flat biotype. The thick flat type is more prevalent (85%) than the thin scalloped biotype (15%).[88,89,90] Each type has morphological characteristics of its own with its distinctive adjoining structures. Recognizing and distinguishing these basic types is essential in selecting the implant size, implant type, and surgical approach, and in predicting the overall prognosis that will result in biological harmony between the dental implants and the existing dentogingival structures.

The thick flat biotype (Figs 2.14a,b) is characterized by adequate amounts of masticatory mucosa. It is dense and fibrous in nature with minimal height difference between the highest and lowest points on the proximal and facial aspects of the marginal gingiva; therefore, it is

width is needed to achieve optimal health of the tissues surrounding natural dentition.[83,84] Others have suggested that less than 1 mm of keratinized tissue can be adequate, provided the bacterial plaque is well controlled.[85]

Generally speaking, the presence of a sufficient band of keratinized mucosa will surely improve the aesthetic outcome of the definitive implant-supported restoration. The presence of the keratinized band can also minimize postoperative gingival recession, endure the trauma of brushing, resist masticatory muscle pull, and reduce the probability of soft tissue dehiscence above implant fixtures. Because soft tissues have the tendency to recede almost 1 mm after surgical and restorative implant procedures,[86] a sufficient amount of healthy keratinized gingival tissue should exist prior to implant placement for compensation. Therefore, optimizing the soft tissue quality and quantity before commencing on implant therapy becomes a vital prerequiste. In the presurgical planning stage, the timing of soft tissue augmentation therapy (whether it is to be performed before, during, or after implant placement) will be determined.

Note that Chapter 4 will cover all the soft tissue manipulations around dental implants.

TISSUE BIOTYPES

Healthy human periodontium is comprised of radicular cementum, periodontal ligament, gingiva, and investing alveolar bone.[87] It is the integration of all these biological elements that maintains the periodontium in a state of harmony that makes it unique. The natural morphology of the healthy periodontium is characterized by a rise and fall of the marginal gingiva following the underlying alveolar crest contour both facially and proximally.

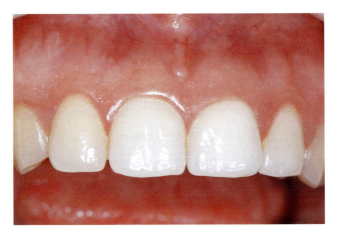

FIGURE 2.14a. Thick flat tissue biotype clinically; note the square shape of the crown and the width of the keratinized tissue band.

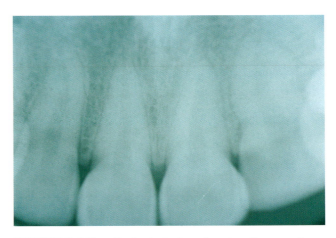

FIGURE 2.14b. Periapical view showing the morphological characters of the thick flat tissue biotype. Note the reduced inter-radicular bone thickness.

called flat. Larger sized teeth that are most likely square shaped characterize this type of periodontium. This bulkiness of the tooth shape results in a broader, more apically positioned contact area, a cervical convexity that has greater prominence, and an embrasure that is completely filled with the interdental papilla. The root dimensions are broader mesiodistally, almost equal to the width of the crown at the cervix, which causes a diminution in the amount of bone interproximally. The typical reaction of this tissue biotype to trauma such as tooth preparation or impression making is inflammation and apical migration of the junctional epithelium with a resultant pocket formation.

The thick flat tissue type is ideal for placing dental implants. Here the gingival and osseous scalloping is normally parallel to the cementoenamel junction (CEJ).[91] The minimal undulation of the CEJ between adjacent teeth, which predictably follows the natural contour of the alveolar crest, makes the gingival tissues more stable. Consequently, this type of periodontium is less likely to exhibit soft tissue shrinkage postoperatively.[91]

On the other hand, the thin scalloped biotype of periodontium exhibits its own distinctive features. These include thin, friable gingiva with a narrow band of attached masticatory mucosa, and a thin facial bone that usually exhibits dehiscence and fenestration (Fig 2.15a,b). The tooth crown shape usually exhibits a triangular or thin cylindrical form, and the contact areas are smaller and located in a further incisal location. The cervical convexity is less prominent than that of the thick biotype, while the interdental papilla is thin and long but does not fill the embrasure space completely, resulting in a scalloped appearance.[92] Additionally, this biotype possesses a root that is narrow with an attenuated taper,

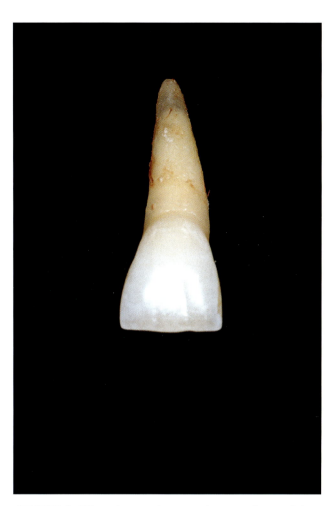

FIGURE 2.15b. A view showing the root shape of the thin scalloped dentition.

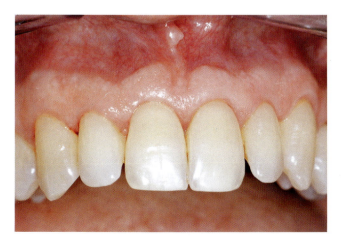

FIGURE 2.15a. Clinical picture of the thin scalloped tissue biotype. Note the reduced crown width and the apically located interdental papillae.

allowing for an increased amount of interradicular bone. When inflicted with trauma, this tissue type undergoes gingival recession both facially and interproximally. Placing dental implants in the aesthetic zone becomes a critical task with this particular tissue biotype because it is difficult to achieve symmetrical soft tissue contours probably due to the proximity of the implant to the natural tooth periodontium next to it, and the reduced amount of masticatory mucosa.[93] The resultant recession and bone resorption leave a flat profile between the roots, with marginal exposure of the restoration and subsequent partial loss of the interproximal papilla.[94]

A proper appraisal of the periodontium should be performed prior to commencing any implant therapy in the aesthetic zone. Each tissue type reacts differently to surgical intervention, thereby warranting a specific treatment protocol. The thin scalloped tissue type should be treated with an exceptional caution and utmost care (especially for patients with a high smile line).

BONE QUANTITY AND QUALITY

Replacing missing dentition with dental implants demands both optimized bone quantity and bone quality at the edentulous site. Optimal osseous volume has a positive influence on osseointegration.[95–97] Therefore, emphasis should be placed on inserting an implant in a sufficient osseous foundation when a predictable, successful aesthetic and functional outcome is to be achieved.

It has been reported that the alveolar bone loses almost 30% of its size within two years following tooth extraction.[98] Both maxilla and mandible have distinctive resorption patterns that affect both the width and height of the alveolar bone (Fig. 2.16).[99–101] Subsequently, bone dimensions become insufficient to host the implant fixture, thus negatively affecting the overall prognosis of the implant-supported prosthesis. It follows that alveolar bone quantity and quality are an absolute necessity for dental implant success on both levels—aesthetically and functionally.

The significance of the quantitative and qualitative parameters of the osseous structure is immense; consequently, the subject has been discussed at length in most textbooks. Many authors have classified the remaining alveolar bone differently in order to assess and diagnose the remaining alveolar bone. Misch has classified the available alveolar bone into four distinct divisions[95]:

Division A (Abundant Bone). Alveolar bone width is more than 5 mm, height greater than 10–13 mm, and mesiodistal length greater than 7 mm, and the load's angulation does not exceed 30 degrees between the occlusal plan and the implant body. In addition, the crown–implant body ratio is less than one. This type

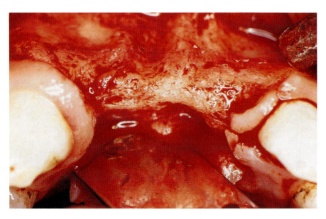

FIGURE 2.16. View of anterior maxilla showing severe bone resorption that hinders implant placement.

of bone is optimal for hosting an implant with a diameter between 4 and 5 mm.

Division B (Barely Sufficient Bone). A slight to moderate atrophy has occurred, leading to a decrease in the width of the available bone at the expense of only the facial cortical bone. The height remains stable at a minimum of 10 mm. The remaining available bone width varies between 3 and 5 mm and is thus able to accommodate an implant of 4 mm maximum width. The load's angulation may not exceed 20 degrees. Treatment options presented for this type are osteoplasty, bone augmentation, or the use of narrower diameter root form dental implants.

Division C (Compromised Bone). Moderate to advanced atrophy is present, with the width less than 2.5 mm, height less than 10 mm, load angulation greater than 30 degrees, and crown–implant body ratio equal to or greater than one. The posterior maxillary and mandibular regions demonstrate this type of alveolar bone more than the anterior segments.

Division D (Deficient Bone). This type demonstrates severe atrophy, accompanied by basal bone loss. Therefore, the use of autogenous bone grafts is strongly recommended to augment the deficient alveolar bone. This kind of bone usually results in complications related to soft tissue management, grafting, and early implant failure.

The above classification can help the practitioner to precisely determine the specific bone category of each particular patient. This, in turn, enables the clinician to select the appropriate treatment protocol. The necessity of undergoing a bone grafting procedure exists in many conditions, and subsequently, a surgical technique can be chosen that provides a treatment prognosis with maximum predictability from either an aesthetic or functional aspect.

Salama and Salama have introduced another classification that considers the available bone according to the socket condition that will host the future implant fixture.[102] This classification can be helpful when an immediate implant placement is the treatment of choice, because the condition of the alveolar socket will dictate the treatment plan. Details of this classification are provided later in this chapter.

Several techniques are now available for evaluation of bone quantity and quality. Radiographic examination, especially tomograms or CT scans, can provide the accurate dimension for the alveolar ridge at a specific predetermined location, as well as the bone density. Bone density in the aesthetic zone generally falls into the D3 category, where 65% of the anterior maxilla constitutes this category.[103]

In many conditions, it is extremely important to assess the bone architecture using a CT scan or a ridge mapping method[29] because the anterior maxilla usually exhibits labial concavities that might necessitate bone grafting procedures or placing the implant fixture at an angle and using a pre-angled abutment.[104]

Reconstruction of the deficient alveolar bone in the aesthetic zone will be discussed in detail in Chapter 5.

ORTHODONTIC AND ENDODONTIC CONSIDERATIONS

The increased demand for the use of dental implants to restore missing dentition and enhance aesthetics has led orthodontics to become an integral part of a multidisciplinary approach to implant therapy. This approach can help solve certain clinical dilemmas and reduce the tendency for performing invasive surgical procedures.

As a result of tooth loss, especially due to premature extraction of deciduous dentition, drifting of the remaining teeth occurs. Therefore, there will be a demand to recreate or develop the lost space to its original optimal dimensions.[105] The use of a narrower implant diameter is not always considered a preferred treatment modality in most of these conditions because narrow implants often result in compromised aesthetic and functional results. Developing space (Fig. 2.17a–e) for the missing dentition therefore becomes valuable in regaining the original natural dimensions.

Salama and Salama[106] were the first to describe the applications of the conventional orthodontic techniques

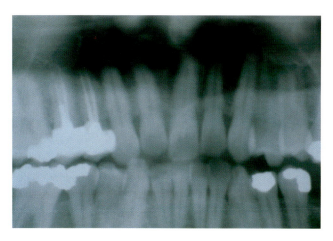

FIGURE 2.17b. Panoramic view confirming the absence of the congenitally missing tooth in the maxillary bone.

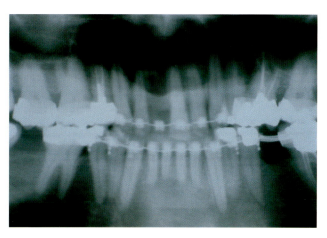

FIGURE 2.17c. Panoramic view showing the space created with orthodontic movement where the upright position of the roots is evident.

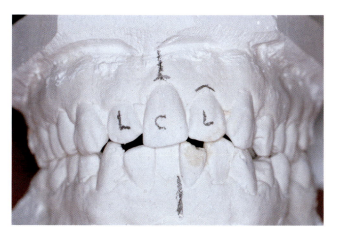

FIGURE 2.17a. A study cast showing a congenitally missing maxillary right central incisor.

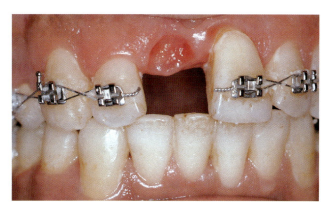

FIGURE 2.17d. The space developed is clinically noticed.

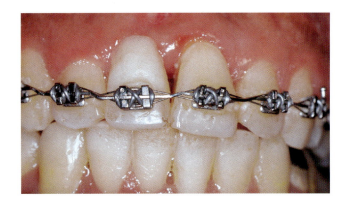

FIGURE 2.17e. A pontic attached to the orthodontic wire to be used as a provisional prosthesis.

to facilitate implant placement.[102] They made use of the so-called restorative orthodontics to develop the supragingival restorative space (space development). They applied this technique in situations where the residual space was not sufficient for placing a dental implant.

In some cases selecting the venue of implants as a treatment of choice must be disregarded. This is especially the case when a space may not be created orthodontically, either because orthodontic treatment is not indicated or because the patient refuses to go through with it.

The periodontic-orthodontic management is yet another clinical treatment approach that has been suggested for achieving greater osseous support.[107,108] This method entails forced eruption of unsalvageable residual roots that will be replaced by dental implants (Fig. 2.18a). In other words, soft and hard tissues may be manipulated to favor the placement of an aesthetic restoration.[109]

Orthodontic extrusive remodeling or extrusion combined with tooth extraction is used currently in regular orthodontic treatments.[102] This procedure is originally performed to gain access to deep carious cavities or in the treatment of crown and root fractures below gingival margins. In this technique, slow eruption of teeth using a light eruptive force of 25–30 g will result in a coronal migration of the entire attachment apparatus.[110] As a result, new bone is deposited in the apical area above the root apex, and is accompanied by an increase in the width of the attached mucosa and the proximal papillae at the cervical area (Fig. 2.18b–k).[111]

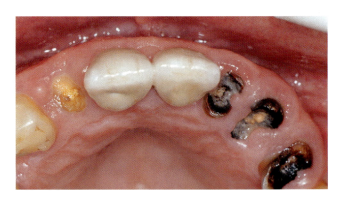

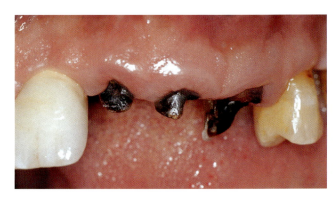

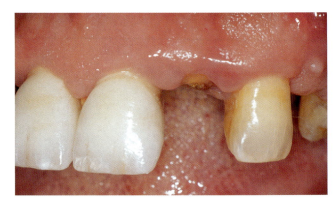

FIGURE 2.18b,c,d. Three different clinical views of unsalvageable severely compromised anterior teeth with loss of the natural height of the interdental papillae.

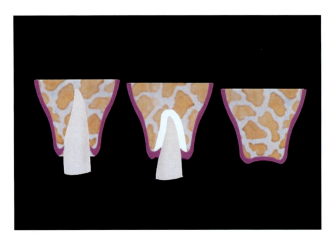

FIGURE 2.18a. Illustration showing forced eruption.

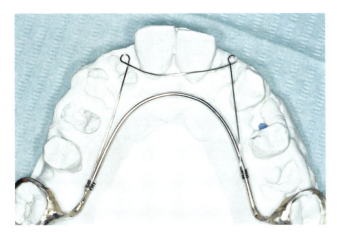

FIGURE 2.18e. Orthodontic appliance on the cast to move the remaining roots in an occlusal direction.

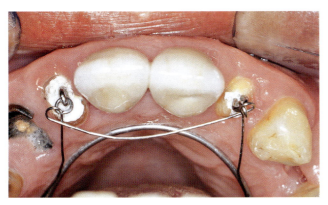

FIGURE 2.18f. The appliance in place; note the hook with the rings attached together.

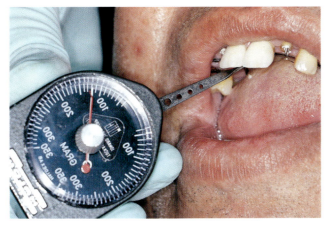

FIGURE 2.18g. A device that measures the optimal force used to activate forced eruption.

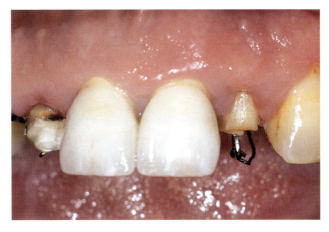

FIGURE 2.18h. Forced eruption occurred to the roots with remarkable movement of the interdental papillae in an incisal direction.

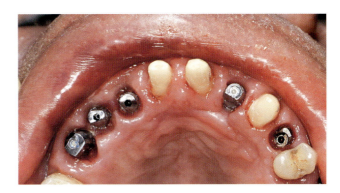

FIGURE 2.18i. Implants in place.

During extrusive orthodontic movement, the alveolar bone attached to the root surface by periodontal fibers migrates along with the investing soft tissues in an incisal direction. Thus, an increase in the available alveolar bone height is to be expected.[112] Subsequently, the coronal migration of the attachment complex promotes regeneration of the papilla and adjacent gingival contours, thus enhancing the aesthetic outcome. The tooth to be removed must be allowed to move only in an axial direction without tipping, which might cause penetration of the labial plate. Extrusion should be brought about at a speed that does not exceed the rate of bone deposition. It usually requires three to four months to occur. This is only half the waiting time needed for a bone-grafting procedure, bearing in mind that this procedure is less traumatic to the patient than others. On the other hand, patient selection and motivation are important factors to be considered before undertaking these procedures.

The local surrounding environment of the proposed implant sites can be an issue of concern during the presurgical stage of implant therapy. Any endodontic lesion should be eliminated before any implant surgery takes place, because it can lead to a possible implant failure.[113] During the initial stage of osseointegration, the

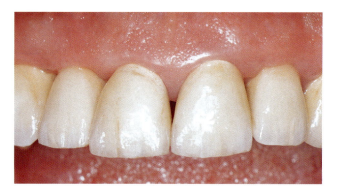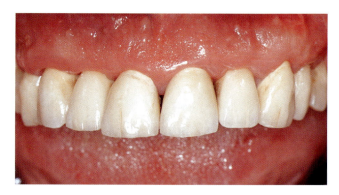

FIGURE 2.18j,k.   The case restored finally.

implant can be particularly vulnerable if placed in closer proximity to an endodontic pathological lesion.[114] This thought was raised in a case report by Sussman in which he suggested that an implant does not have the ability to withstand any bacterial challenge during the healing period.[115]

However, Novaes and Novaes[116] later argued that placement of an implant into a socket that has a chronic endodontic lesion does not necessarily result in failure, provided certain precautions are taken.[116] The authors suggested complete removal of the causative factor (the unsalvageable tooth) with careful and thorough debridement of the socket. Administration of antibiotics to begin at least two days prior to surgery and to be maintained ten days postoperatively was recommended. This was intended to reduce or eliminate the likelihood of bacterial contamination; after the course of antibiotics was completed the host cells could take control. The decision whether to remove the lesion before or with the implant placement remains dependent on the clinician's judgment.

FACIAL ANALYSIS

Patients electing to go through aesthetic reconstructive surgery have certain expectations. These expectations revolve around an improvement in the way they look, specifically their smile; patients focus not particularly on the new restoration itself as a separate entity, but rather on what it has done for their final overall appearance.[117] Therefore, the smile is considered a major component that should be involved in the presurgical evaluation and should be emphasized in any aesthetic treatment plan.

For any aesthetic reconstruction of the oral cavity to be regarded as being comprehensive in nature, an indepth analysis of the facial morphology and structures is mandatory to ensure a harmonious treatment outcome. The facial structures that are considered integral to the examination, as related to the dental assembly, are the lip

anatomy, lip line, lip curvature, nasolabial angle, lip thickness, smile line, and facial complexion.

The outline of the lip, or lip-frame, that surrounds natural dentition is a major facial element that contributes dramatically to dental aesthetics; consequently, it demands careful inspection.[118] Several authors have described the anatomical landmarks of the lip in order to diagnose facial deformities and assist in defining an optimal treatment plan (Fig. 2.19); the Burstone line is a reference line that connects the subnasale point to the pogonion point. The upper and lower lips are compressed by this reference line (ideally +3.5 and +2.2 mm, respectively, above this line).[119] The Steiner line is a line joining the midpoint of the nose to the chin, where the patent's lips touch this line.[120] The Ricketts' E-plane describes a line that extends from the tip of the nose to the chin, in which the maxillary and mandibular lip positions measure 4 and 2 mm, respectively.[121] For the most favorable facial aesthetics, the distance between the subnasale point (base of the nose) and the upper lip should be approximately half the distance measured from the lower lip to the menton (lowest chin) point.[122]

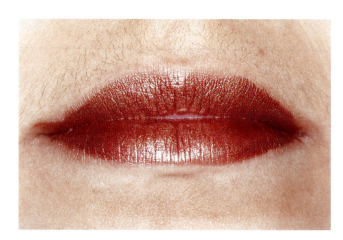

FIGURE 2.19.   Lip anatomy.

Lip size and thickness may sometimes influence the aesthetic perspective of the patient, and consequently, the treatment plan to be embarked upon. It is the author's opinion that a thick lip can mask the marginal artifacts of the final prosthesis to some extent, and it can also influence the restoration design. (Fig. 2.20). On the other hand, a patient with a thin lip tends to exhibit a greater display of the entire restoration, which in most cases has lingually inclined margins. Additionally, the thinner the lip, the shorter the tooth and more lingual its position.[123] Therefore, careful evaluation of lip size, thickness, and character will define what shape and form the future restoration should have. At the same time, it will determine how much of the restoration should be displayed while smiling or with the lip in any other position.

The teeth and the alveolar bone support the outward position of the lips. Once loss of dentition has occurred, it is followed by typical bone resorption on the facial aspect of the maxilla. As a result, the lip loses its support and tonicity, and appears wrinkled or dropped or sunken in (Fig. 2.21a,b). To regain the original state of the lip's tone, dental implants should be placed at the original site of the missing tooth to be replaced and not where the bone is available. A carefully fabricated wax-up on the study cast will indicate the amount of osseous structure required facially to support the lip and return it to its original position. Note that the cervical and middle thirds of the crown contour are to a great extent mostly responsible for determining the lip support.[124]

Changes in the facial musculature that occur as a result of the incumbent emotional state lead to the smile effect. It is the manner in which the lips, teeth, and silhouettes blend to create harmony that gives a smile its own unique magical character.[125] The profound psychological effect that smiling has on a human being explains its value.[126] The development of the smile, from the quar-

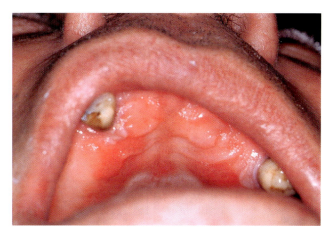

FIGURE 2.21a. A view showing missing anterior teeth that led to drop of the lip, due to losing its support.

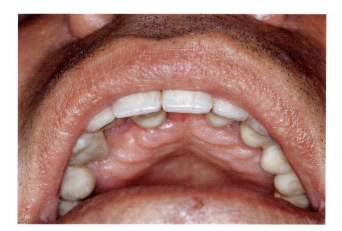

FIGURE 2.21b. The lip support is restored after comprehensive oral reconstruction.

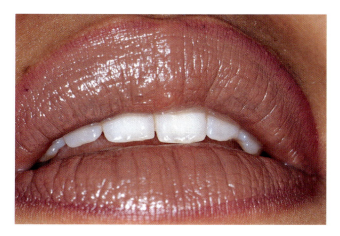

FIGURE 2.20. Thick lip can mask many prosthetic artifacts.

ter smile, to the half smile, to the full smile, in relation to the amount of tooth displayed will suggest to the clinician whether to display or hide the morphological deviation in tooth-gingival relationships.[127] A smile line is defined by Philips as a line that shows a dark or negative space when both jaws separate (Fig. 2.22a–c).[128] In other words, the silhouettes of the incisal edges of the maxillary teeth in comparison to the mandibular incisal edges can also define the smile line.

In young individuals, only 3–4 mm of the incisal edges of the maxillary central incisors are usually displayed at the rest or repose position of the lips. With a full smile, the maxillary lip is required to translate approximately 6–8 mm to expose almost 10–11 mm of the clinical crown. A patient with a hyperactive maxillary lip, however, may translate 1.5–2 times the normal distance.[131] In older patients the upper lip loses its muscle tone and

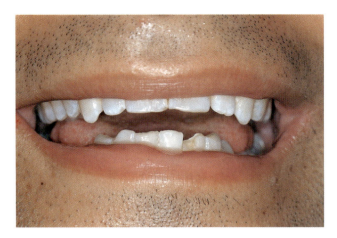

FIGURE 2.22a. Low smile line.

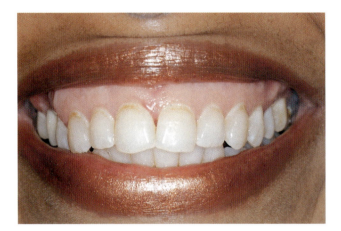

FIGURE 2.22b. High smile line.

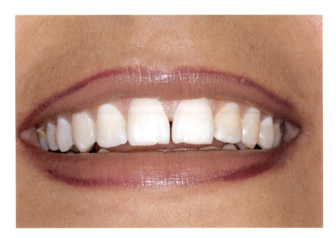

FIGURE 2.22c. Medium smile line.

tends to lengthen, hiding more of the maxillary dentition and exposing more of the mandibular dentition; this observation can be valuable when a totally edentulous patient is to receive restorative rehabilitative treatment.

Rubin has classified smiles into five categories: a maxillary smile showing only the maxillary teeth; a maxillary smile showing more than 3 mm of gingiva, also often referred to as a gummy smile; a solely mandibular smile; a smile with both maxillary and mandibular teeth appearing; and lastly, a smile which is neither maxillary nor mandibular.[129] It is noteworthy to mention that a gummy smile or an increased bite overjet does not necessarily warrant reconstructive correction. Sometimes, if the gingival tissue that is exposed during a smile is moderate, it can add a touch of beauty to the facial complex, thereby giving a distinctive appearance to the person (Fig. 2.23).

Rubin also stated that there are three basic styles of smiles. A commissure smile is the most common type (67%); the corners of the mouth are initially pulled upward and outward, followed by rising of the upper lip to exhibit only the maxillary teeth. A cupid smile, occur-

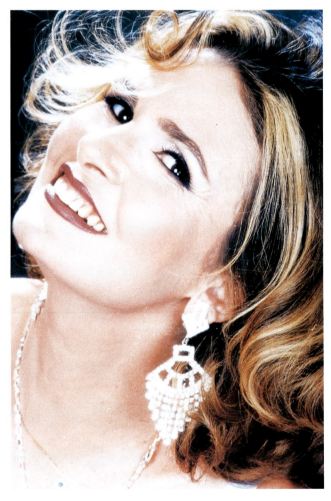

FIGURE 2.23. A picture of a famous Egyptian actress showing a slight gingival display that can add to the beauty of the face.

ring in 31% of the population, exposes the canines and then the corners of the mouth. A complex smile, however, appears in only 2% of the population; it shows all the maxillary and mandibular teeth simultaneously during elevation of the upper lip and contraction of the lower lip.[129]

Smile design is a novel expression introduced by Morley.[130] He defined smile design as a discipline involving the diagnosis and subsequent planning for primarily the aesthetic component of the overall dental treatment. In other words, it is the modification of the amount of tooth displayed while smiling, using the available tools and applying the principles of design to anterior dental aesthetics. This approach can turn an average restorative job into an outstanding one while at the same time preserving the existing natural beauty.[131]

Aesthetic factors that contribute to smile design and can be influenced in the treatment consist of the incisal and occlusal plane; size and inclination of the central incisors; midline position; axial alignment of the remaining teeth; size and form of the arch; lip line to the incisal edge position; form and morphology of the dentition; position of the contact points; and gingival height, zenith color, and contour.[136–138]

The maxillary central incisors play an important role in smile design. They represent the gateway to the oral cavity and are invariably apparent in any smile. It is no wonder that a missing central incisor is best restored when a method that focuses on duplicating the original natural tooth's appearance is selected. Therefore, information about the original position, shape, and size of the central incisors is vital to restoring a patient's smile.[132] Moreover, in major aesthetic reconstructive procedures, it is important that the midline be adjusted centrally to coordinate with the other anatomical landmarks in the face, to obtain complete harmony of the dentofacial complex.[133–135]

The shape of the central incisors can arbitrarily reveal a patient's age or gender. A longer, rectangular-shaped central incisor, gives a more youthful appearance.[133] On the other hand, incisal wear and attrition that occur with age result in a short and square central incisor, which characterizes old age. Lateral incisors can reveal the gender of a person. A feminine lateral incisor possesses a more constricted neck with rounded incisal edges, while masculine lateral incisors tend to be flatter and wider, with square incisoproximal angles, and sometimes attain a width closer to that of the neighboring central incisors (Fig. 2.24a,b).[133,134]

All these observations should be gathered from range of facial expressions as well as during various forms of the patient's speech. Since individuals are conditioned to conceal aesthetic discrepancies with pretentious rather than natural demeanors, these extreme facial expressions or poses must be carefully recorded before the treatment commences.[135]

EMERGENCE PROFILE

The ability of the clinician to understand and control the relationship between the implant and its associated gingival structures is extremely important in achieving an aesthetic final implant-supported restoration. The position of the gingival margin following stage-two surgery represents a collapsed state, until it finds support by the prosthetic components against which it comes to rest.[111] The gingival tissues around dental implant components should be enhanced, influenced and developed to acquire the same dimensions and configurations as the original

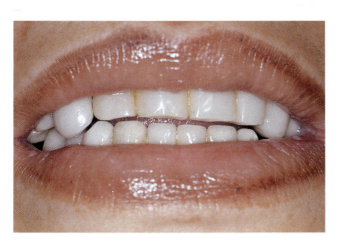

FIGURE 2.24a. Showing an unpleasant smile due to improper position and morphology of the prosthesis.

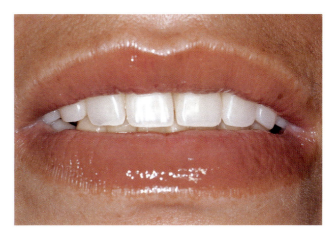

FIGURE 2.24b. Showing the remarkable improvement of the smile after replicating the original tooth form and position.

tissues around natural dentition. The original soft tissue configuration around natural teeth possesses a flat profile at the point where they erupt from the marginal mucosa (Fig. 2.25).[139,140]

The use of the different prosthetic components after the second-stage surgery will allow the maturation of peri-implant soft tissue to develop a peri-implant dimension in the subgingival area that gradually develops the emergence profile of the final prosthesis matching the dimensions of the tooth to be replicated. The use of an accurately fabricated surgical template can help ensure accurate implant positioning in relation to the adjacent dentition, which directly influences the resultant emergence profile.[141] Therefore, precise implant placement and careful soft-tissue manipulation will allow the clinician to enhance the peri-implant soft-tissue contours with the use of provisional restorations. Provisional restoration will encourage gingival maturation to provide an ideal frame for the implant-supported prosthesis. The cervical third of the labial aspect of the provisional prosthesis is responsible for stimulating peri-implant tissues and developing the natural emergence. The basic requirements for successful guided provisional soft-tissue modeling are sufficient keratinized gingiva, provisional abutments, gradual atraumatic provisionalization, and realistic size of the amount of gingival expansion.

Achieving a flat emergence profile around implant-supported prostheses warrants obtaining sufficient information on the specific tissue biotype, tooth form, soft tissue health condition, adjacent periodontal health

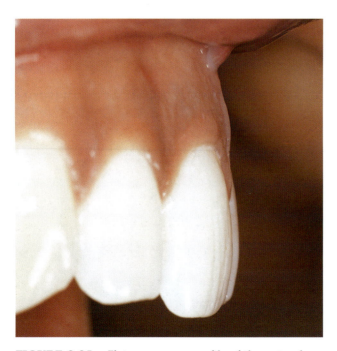

FIGURE 2.25. Flat emergence profile of the natural maxillary anterior teeth.

condition, and the type of future prosthetic components to be used. Since an implant differs from a natural tooth in its morphological characteristics, the cylindrical shape of the implant has to be improved upon in the subgingival compartment. It rarely corresponds to that of a tooth. This compels the clinician to compensate for this discrepancy by developing the soft tissue through the precise fabrication of a provisional restoration that transfers the cylindrical shape of the implant to the shape of the root of the natural tooth at the gingival margin, that gradually influences the peri-implant soft tissue to the desired configuration.[142]

SURGICAL TEMPLATE

Optimal placement of dental implants becomes a vital clinical prerequisite in fulfilling the patient's desires and expectations.[143] The precise placement of dental implants is essential to designing a prosthesis that satisfies the aesthetic and functional requirements and simultaneously allows clear phonetics and facilitates oral hygiene.

Prosthetic-driven implant placement is the golden rule that ensures predictable treatment results. Thus, transfer of the information regarding optimal position and angulation for the implant fixture from the study cast onto the surgical site becomes mandatory. A precisely fabricated surgical template or guide has an active role in executing the treatment plan at the first stage of surgery and determining the position of the implants at the second-stage surgery. Furthermore, this presurgical step in implant treatment aids in the preservation of the required biological space between the implant and the neighboring roots. Besides that, it assists in keeping the recommended distance between implant fixtures themselves. All of these advantages ultimately assist in an increase in the precision of aesthetic implant positioning and an improved final outcome of the prosthesis.

Several factors must be taken into consideration before deciding on the design of the future template to be used. These encompass the future implant position, number of implants to be used, the existing occlusion, the amount of available bone, the soft tissue status, the type of implant prosthetic components, and the type of future definitive prosthesis.[144]

The basic simplest surgical template is fabricated from a clear resin duplicate of the diagnostic wax-up. It has guiding grooves or cutouts at the location of the potential implant sites. These are usually fabricated according to the original position of the missing dentition; the exact amount of hard and soft tissue that should be regenerated to provide a healthy biological contour will be automatically identified after the template construction.[145] The template is placed on the working cast, and drill holes of 3 mm diameter are prepared through the cingula of the anterior teeth and/or on the center of the occlusal surfaces of posterior teeth.[146] These guide holes will be used to guide the pilot drill in the bone.

Most fabricated surgical templates are limited to two planes, excluding the apicoincisal plane of the implant.[147] However, there are available surgical templates that can also be used to indicate the distance required to countersink the implant. This is accomplished by making room for a gradual emergence from the relatively narrow implant platform to the comparatively wide cervical portion of the restoration.[92,148] The greater the accuracy of the surgical template fabrication, the more precise the implant positioning obtained.

The design of the surgical template differs according to the complexity of the case. In partially edentulous cases, where the edentulous area is bounded by remaining dentition, the template need not be extended anteroposteriorly more than two teeth on each side of the edentulous space and can be trimmed accordingly.[146]

The commonly used surgical template can either be a partial denture with indented markings on the acrylic teeth indicating the site of the future implants (with palatal or lingual relief) or a transparent template with a guiding hole that allows the drill to penetrate into the bone.[149,150] Both types lack precise implant positioning because the template does not provide a control for the buccolingual movement of the drill. For that reason, any deviation in the direction of the drilling angulation will subsequently alter the future implant position (Fig. 2.26). A panoramic radiograph can be taken with the surgical template in place to help determine the best location and angulation of implants relative to the proposed prosthesis.[35] Radiopaque ball bearings of a known diameter are luted into the template and appear suspended over potential implant placement sites on the radiograph. By dividing the actual diameter of the ball bearing by the diameter of its image on the radiograph, the distortion

factor of the panoramic image can be calculated for each proposed implant location.[35] The actual height of the residual ridge can then be calculated by multiplying the distortion factor by the distance from the crest of the ridge to any anatomical landmark. This procedure assists in the selection of accurate implant length. After radiographic diagnosis is made, the ball bearings are removed and the template is perforated and sterilized to be used during the implant surgery.[35]

Another advanced technique used to construct a precise surgical template is integration of a stainless steel sleeve into the acrylic resin body of the template around the drill hole.[151,152] This type of template permits exact implant positioning with accurate parallelism. The sleeves help maintain parallel holes throughout the drilling procedure; they also prevent the acrylic resin from being distorted or chipped off at the surgical site (from the sharp friction of the surgical drill with the sides of the template). Presence of the sleeves provides a stable position for the drill and fixed angulation throughout the drilling procedure (Fig. 2.27a–c).

A dual-purpose template is another precise surgical template that maintains a correct labiopalatal position of dental implants.[153] It offers not only precise information about the location and angulation of the implant but also, subsequent to a tomographic evaluation, information on the anticipated abutment relative to the predesigned suprastructure.[154]

Recently, the terms *computer-guided surgery* and *computer-milled surgical templates* have been introduced.[155] The computer-milled surgical template (Compu-surge Template, Implant Logic Systems, Cedarhurst, New York, U.S.A.) provides a connection between the CT scan

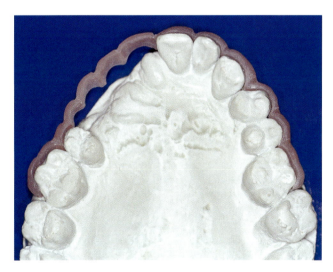

FIGURE 2.27a. The acrylic template can show the amount of bone to be regenerated to regain the original contours.

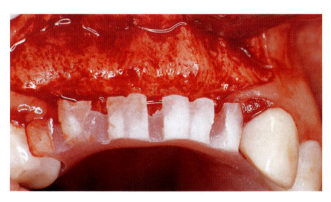

FIGURE 2.26. The commonly used surgical template that has guiding grooves lacks axial control of the drill.

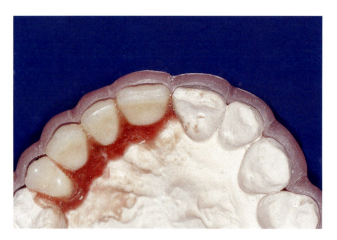

FIGURE 2.27b. Wax-up of the case.

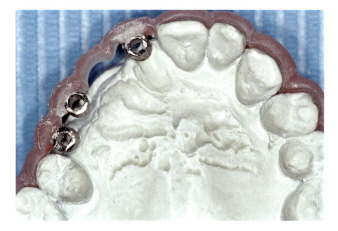

FIGURE 2.27c. The stainless steel sleeves are attached to the acrylic template for accurate implant positioning.

and the surgical template. It utilizes reformatted CT data in combination with a three-dimensional simulation of the implant position to produce a computer-milled surgical template. The simulated implant position is created via SIM/Plant software (SIM/Plant, Columbia Scientific, Columbia, Maryland, U.S.A.). The three-dimensional coordinates of the simulated implant position will be transferred to a five-axis computer-controlled milling machine that creates an appliance with the SIM/Plant plan. Drill guide components are then installed in the milled surgical template to direct the drilling procedure.

The Novel guide template is one of the most recently introduced surgical templates that eliminates the problem of template slippage on the flap. With no slippage, the risk of plastic or metal debris from the template entering into the wound is eliminated because the template itself does not have an active role in the drilling procedure. This guide template is best used when placing multiple

implants.[156] It is fabricated from the wax-up on the diagnostic cast. Precise determination of the implant angulation is obtained by providing a guide sleeve on the 0.8 mm Kirschner wires within the template. The template is placed in position over the intact mucosa surface. The template guides the Kirschner wires to pierce through the mucosa into the bone. The wires are attached to a special insert using a dental coupling fitted into the dental handpiece. The insert facilitates easy insertion of the wires into the bone. The wires are then trimmed 5–7 mm above the bone level; then incisions are made to connect the wires to each other or to the adjacent natural tooth. After the insertion of the wires, the implant osteotomies are prepared with a trephine drill guided over the wires alone or over wires combined with a special guidance cylinder fitting the trephine drill (Fig. 2.28a–e). This method may alleviate some of the problems common to conventional

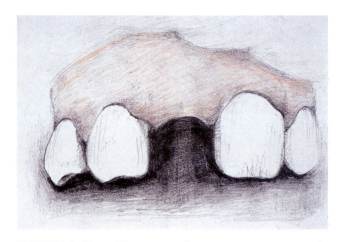

FIGURE 2.28a. Illustration showing a missing central incisor.

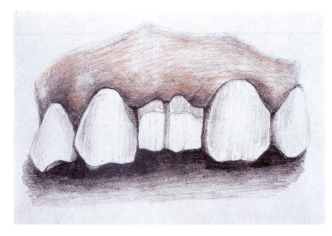

FIGURE 2.28b. The Novel guide is put in the place of the missing tooth.

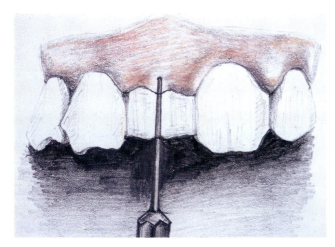

FIGURE 2.28c. The Kirschner wire being introduced through the mucosa.

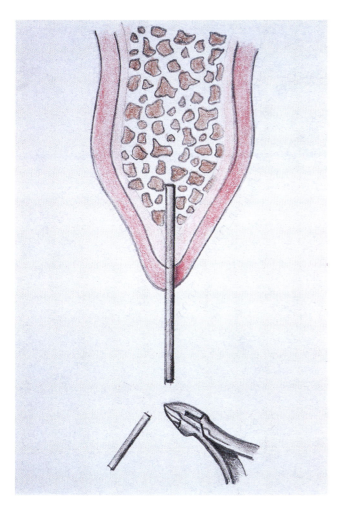

FIGURE 2.28d. The wire trimmed off.

template techniques, where the template usually directly guides the drill, whereas the guiding wires allow for precise implant positioning in the alveolar ridge.

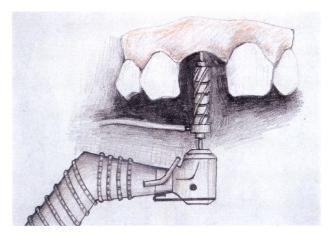

FIGURE 2.28e. The remaining Kirschner wire is the guide for the trephine drill. Note that in using the Novel guide, the pilot drill is replaced with a small-diameter trephine drill.

PLANNING FOR SURGICAL INTERVENTION

Appropriate timing of the implant placement in the alveolar ridge is essential. It can influence aesthetic soft tissue contours around dental implants, especially when the anterior maxilla is concerned.

The decision whether to insert the implant immediately upon unsalvageable tooth extraction or to delay its placement until complete socket healing occurs is based on many factors.[157] These determining factors include soft tissue health and integrity, tissue biotype, the need for preservation of interdental papillae, prevention of the alveolar ridge resorption, the pathological and morphological condition of the alveolar socket immediately after extraction, patient demands, and the predictability of osseointegration. It must be duly noted that the decision on the timing of dental implant placement is critical and can significantly affect treatment results from the aesthetic standpoint and/or that of serviceability.

The standard protocol for placing dental implants requires an alveolar ridge that is completely healed before inserting the implant fixture.[158] It is called the delayed implant placement protocol and requires a healing period varying between five and nine months post–tooth extraction before implant placement.[80] The healing period not only allows the placement of the implant fixture in mature osseous architecture, but also permits the maturation of the associated soft tissue in the future implant site. This ultimately minimizes the need for excessive soft tissue manipulative procedures required to achieve primary soft tissue closure (Fig. 2.29a–c). The need for bone grafting procedures is also minimized especially in the posterior areas because greater implant-bone contact is ensured.

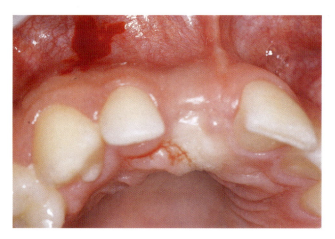

FIGURE 2.29a. Six months postextraction allowing for delayed implant placement.

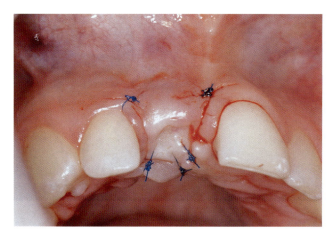

FIGURE 2.29b. The implant inserted and the flap closed without any soft tissue modification procedure in delayed implant placement.

This in turn eliminates the possibility of epithelial downgrowth into the osteotomy site. However, delayed implant placement may not be the treatment of choice in all regions. In the maxillary anterior zone, in particular, delaying implant placement results in alveolar ridge resorption, both in the buccolingual and apicoincisal directions,[159] which usually necessitates the use of guided tissue regenerative techniques, in order to maintain maximum aesthetics. Furthermore, studies have shown that as much as 3–4 mm of alveolar ridge resorption can occur during the first six months after tooth extraction (if no bone-grafting procedures have been performed at the time of tooth extraction).[160] Other reports have indicated that 23% of the anterior alveolar ridge resorption takes place within the first six months following tooth extraction.[161] This process significantly affects the topography of the hard and soft tissues, which in turn may hinder the aesthetic three-dimensional positioning of the implant (Fig. 2.30).

Some clinicians, for more than one reason, prefer the delayed implant placement technique. These reasons include reducing the risk of infection and reducing soft tissue manipulations.[179] Postextraction bone resorption remains as an issue of controversy to be reckoned with.

Immediate implant placement has been extensively documented in the literature.[162–164] In this approach, the implant fixture is inserted immediately following the unsalvageable tooth extraction. This procedure may be performed with or without bone grafting of the space between the implant body and the alveolar socket walls. Immediate implant insertion can be an effective method to prevent the alveolus from undergoing postextraction resorption.[165,166]

Several studies have shown success rates using immediate implants comparable to those of implants inserted into healed sites.[167–169] However, there are some prevailing conditions that increased this technique's credibility;

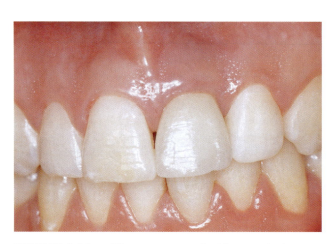

FIGURE 2.29c. The case restored with no soft tissue compromise.

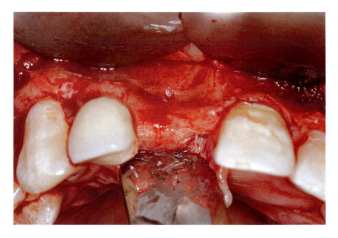

FIGURE 2.30. Two years postextraction bone resorption.

these include absence of infection, good mechanical anchorage and primary stability of the implant fixture, atraumatic removal of the unsalvageable tooth with preservation of the labial plate of bone, use of the appropriate implant size and design that corresponds to the socket's configuration, and proper implant placement in terms of angulation and position. Unfortunately, most of the studies have measured success in terms of osseointegration, but have not considered soft tissue changes. The soft tissue compromise resulting from the attempt to achieve primary closure on top of the socket is the only primary concern that directly influences the final aesthetic results. A recent study recommended the use of wide-diameter implants with caution in aesthetically demanding areas.[170] This was based on the conclusion that after the second stage of surgery the soft tissue recedes around wide-diameter implants an average of 1.58 mm, compared with 0.57 mm around small-diameter implants (Fig. 2.31a–d).[170] Therefore, the use of the wide-diameter implants should be approached with caution in the case of the immediate aesthetic implant placement protocol.

Extraction of a tooth leaves behind a socket that has its own characteristics. Many authors have classified extraction sites at the time of implant placement and

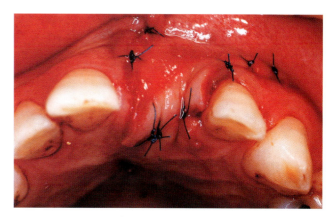

FIGURE 2.31c.   The soft tissue modified to allow for complete closure.

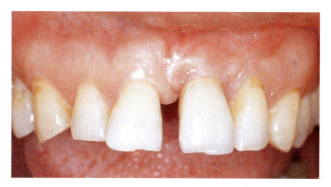

FIGURE 2.31d.   The case restored with some scar tissue formation due to excessive soft tissue manipulations.

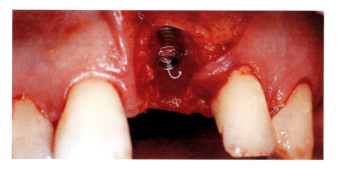

FIGURE 2.31a.   Immediate implant placement.

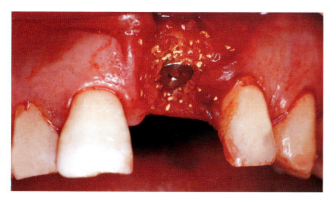

FIGURE 2.31b.   The area is grafted with demineralized freeze-dried bone (DMDB) combined with tetracycline powder.

have suggested clinical solutions for each class.[102,171–175] The classifications of the socket condition can provide the clinician with an accurate diagnostic tool to deal with the different clinical situations. Salama and Salama have classified the socket state into three individual classes[102]: Class One describes a socket that has intact walls and is favorable for immediate implant placement with or without bone grafting. Class Two has a socket with a missing labial wall, necessitating the use of guided tissue regeneration (GTR) and a bone graft in conjunction with implant placement. Class Three refers to a socket that does not provide any implant anchorage and requires the application of a staged implant insertion as well as bone-grafting procedures.

Garber and Belser have categorized immediate implant sites after tooth extraction into three different classes.[173] Their classification was as follows: Type I is a socket having dehiscence of less than 5 mm; this type is almost equivalent to the first class in Salama and Salama's classifications. A Type II socket has a dehiscence equal to 5 mm; it requires autogenous bone grafting and GTR. Type III is a socket with a dehiscence of more than

5 mm; it offers no primary stability for the implant fixture and warrants a staged approach for implant insertion and bone-grafting procedures.

Meltzer described four classes of socket conditions[174]: A Class I socket possesses intact walls all over. A Class II socket has a fenestrated wall. A Class III socket has sufficient bone height, but not enough width, or has two missing osseous walls. Class IV describes a socket with insufficient or no vertical dimension.

A recent classification included, in addition to a three-dimensional classification for the osseous defect, the status of the soft tissues surrounding the immediate dental implants. This classification yields a more accurate description of the status of the socket at the time of immediate implant placement.[175]

The advantages an immediate implant procedure offers are many. They include optimal implant placement (i.e., the original tooth place), which thus minimizes the need for severely angulated abutments, and alveolar ridge preservation due to prevention of the postextraction resorption, which permits the use of longer and wider implants. Other advantages are (1) minimizing the possibility for injury of anatomical landmarks, (2) limiting postdrilling bone resorption by reducing heat generation during drilling, and (3) reducing treatment time to almost half. Additionally, there is a positive psychological impact on the patient in relation to dental implants since immediate replacement of the extracted root/tooth takes place without the patient going through a lapse waiting for socket healing.

Methods of soft tissue closure for immediate implant placement will be explained in detail in Chapter 4.

A nonsubmerged protocol for immediate implantation was proposed.[176] In this protocol, the implant and healing abutment are connected at the time of implant placement without attempting any soft tissue modifications. This technique minimizes soft tissue trauma and plays a significant role in the maturation of the soft tissue around the site. Using an implant diameter that corresponds to the socket orifice will eventually reduce the need for bone grafting and prevent the in-growth of soft tissue along the socket walls.[177] On the other hand, soft tissue closure is still a questionable guarantee for long-term osseointegration. Lack of direct visibility of the labial plate of the alveolar bone raises some serious concerns over this procedure and its clinical success.

The immediate delayed protocol of implant placement, on the other hand, permits soft tissue granulation on the socket orifice. It takes six to ten weeks after tooth extraction to mature. This approach aids in developing a soft tissue seal on top of the socket by secondary intention, after which the implant is placed, as is the case of the standard delayed method. The newly formed keratinized tissue helps minimize soft tissue complications that might arise from excessive surgical manipulations

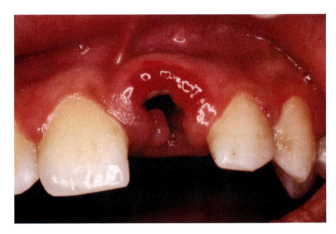

FIGURE 2.32a. Unsalvageable remaining root that will be extracted for implant placement.

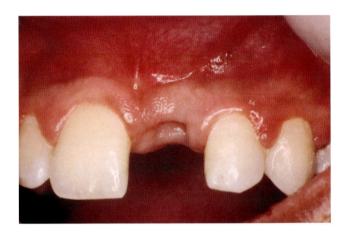

FIGURE 2.32b. Eight weeks after extraction; note the soft tissue closure.

made to achieve primary closure in immediate implant placement cases (Fig. 2.32a,b).

Interestingly, a study described another method for delayed implantation.[178] This technique employs an implant osteotomy followed by wound closure without actually inserting the implant. Two weeks later, the patient undergoes another surgery to place the implant. The authors found that many new thin trabeculae and capillaries formed around the osteotomy walls during the waiting period, and the surrounding fibrous tissue encapsulation appeared to a lesser extent, thus enhancing osseointegration. This approach makes the technique clinically and practically inapplicable.

The one-stage implant placement technique is another implant placement protocol; it refers to the insertion of a one-piece implant in a single surgical procedure, eliminating the second-stage surgery. The technique is similar to the nonsubmerged protocol of implant placement. The implant penetrates the soft tissue through the flared implant neck itself. The method can be used in delayed and immediate cases. The use of nonsubmerged, one-piece implants has shown immense clinical success, especially at the functional level, with the ease of prosthetic management.[180,181] The one-stage system eliminates the possibility of microgap formation between the abutment and the implant fixture at the level of the bone crest. While these advantages certainly increase the popularity of this type of implant, it must be noted that the technique must be restricted to areas where aesthetics are not of chief concern.[182]

Selecting a particular method of implantation will remain the clinician's decision to make after the required presurgical investigations are made.

ARE FUNCTION AND AESTHETICS SEPARABLE?

Restoring function is the primary goal of oral implantology. In the presurgical planning stage, the functional aspect of the implant-supported prostheses should be emphasized and predicted first because dental implants should be placed for long-term survival, and aesthetics come after as a complementary clinical benefit. Any planned implant-supported restorations in the aesthetic zone should fulfill both functional and aesthetic goals, but function should not be jeopardized due to overemphasizing aesthetics, because the priority should be for function. Any aesthetic implant-supported restoration that fails to meet the functional goal cannot be considered a success and vice versa. The delicate balance between function and aesthetics must be maintained because they both complement the treatment outcome, which emphasizes the value of the presurgical stage as an integral part of the treatment.

We, as clinicians, should focus on the full spectrum of oral rehabilitation, which includes both aesthetics and function. Misch stated, "too often the profession concentrates only on aesthetics and soft tissue contours, [which] might be accomplished at the expense of the sulcular health."[183] Therefore, any excess manipulations that focus only on the soft tissue appearance regardless of the osseous support will be disqualified. In other words, solid criteria for patient selection, aseptic surgical techniques, biomechanical concepts, and rigorous maintenance should be carefully regarded in any definitive treatment plan. The ultimate standard for measuring implant success should be the available criteria of Zarb and Schmitt.[82] This will provide patients with an optimum prognosis for long-term rehabilitation.

REFERENCES

1. Malamed SF. Physical and psychological evaluation. In Malamed SF, ed. Sedation: A Guide to Patient Management, 3rd ed. St. Louis: Mosby, 1995, 32–62.
2. Sabes WR, Green S, and Craine C. Value of medical diagnostic screening tests for dental patients. J Am Dent Assoc 1970(80): 133–136.
3. Halstead C, ed. Physical Evaluation of the Dental Patient. St. Louis: Mosby, 1982, 74–81
4. Misch CE. Medical evaluation of the implant candidate. Part II. Int J Oral Implant 1982(2): 11–18.
5. Little JW and Falace DA, eds. Dental Management of the Medically Compromised Patient, 4th ed. St Louis: Mosby, 1993.
6. Matukas VJ. Medical risks associated with dental implants. J Dent Educ 1988(52): 745–747.
7. Smiler DG. Evaluation and treatment planning. J Calif Dent Assoc 1987(10): 35–41.
8. Rees TD, Liverett DM, and Guy CL. The effect of cigarette smoking on skin-flap survival in the face lift patient. Plast Reconstr Surg 1984(73): 911–915.
9. Bergström J and Preber H. Tobacco as a risk factor. J Periodontol 1994 65(May suppl.): 545–550.
10. Grossi SG, Zambon J, Machtei EE, Schifferle R, Adreana S, Genco RJ, Cummins D, Harrap G, et al. Effects of smoking and smoking cessation on healing after mechanical periodontal therapy. J Am Dent Assoc 1997(128): 599–607.
11. Bain CA and Moy PK. The association between the failure of dental implants and cigarette smoking. Int J Oral Maxillofac Implants 1993(8): 609–615.
12. Gorman LM, Lambert PM, Morris HF, Ochi S, Winkler S. The effect of smoking on implant survival at second-stage surgery: DICRG interim report no. 5. Implant Dent 1994(3): 165–168.
13. De Bruyn H and Collaert B. The effect of smoking on early implant failure. Clin Oral Impl Res 1994(5): 260–264.
14. Bain CA. Smoking and implant failure—A smoking cessation protocol. Int J Oral Maxillofac Implants 1996 11(6): 756–759.
15. Williams DF. Titanium as a metal for implantation. Part 2: Biological properties and clinical applications. J Med Eng Tech 1977(9): 266–270.
16. Lekholm U, Adell R, and Brånemark P-I. Complications. In Brånemark P-I, Zarb GA, and Albrektsson T, eds. Tissue-integrated Prostheses. Osseointegration in Clinical Dentistry. Chicago: Quintessence, 1985, 233–240.
17. Latta GH, Jr., McDougal S, and Bowles WF. Response of known nickel-sensitive patient to a removable partial denture with a titanium alloy framework: A clinical report. J Prosthet Dent 1993(70): 109–110.
18. Bezzon OL. Allergic sensitivity to several base metals: A clinical report. J Prosthet Dent 1993(69): 243–244.
19. Hansen PA and West LA. Allergic reaction following insertion of a Pd-Cu-Au fixed partial denture: A clinical report. J Prosthod 1997(6): 144–148.
20. Fielding AF and Hild ER. Maintaining the quality of life in the HIV patient through osseointegrated implants. Abstract. Second International Workshop on the Oral Manifestations of HIV Infection. San Francisco, Jan. 31–Feb. 3, 1993.
21. Melamed BG. Psychological considerations for implant patients. J Oral Implantol 1989 15(4): 249–254.

22. Smith RA, Silverman S, Jr., and Auclert O. Recognition of malignancy and dysplasia in the dental implant patient. J Oral Implantol 1989 15(4): 255—258.

23. Misch EC. Diagnostic casts, preimplant prosthodontics, treatment prostheses, and surgical templates. In Misch CE, ed. Contemporary Implant Dentistry, St. Louis: Mosby, 1999, 135–149.

24. Jovanovic SA. Bone rehabilitation to achieve optimal aesthetics. Pract Periodont Aesthet Dent 1997 9(1): 41–52.

25. Lai JY and Birek P. A simple post-extraction technique for the preservation of the soft tissue architecture leading to a favorable cosmetic outcome for implant prosthetics. Oral Health 1999(89): 19–21.

26. Spear FM. Maintenance of the interdental papilla following anterior tooth removal. Pract Periodont Aesthet Dent 1999 11(1): 21–28.

27. Chiche GJ and Aoshima H. Functional versus aesthetic articulation of maxillary anterior restorations. Pract Periodont Aesthet Dent 1997 9(3): 335–342.

28. Spiekerman HS. Special diagnostic methods for implant patients. In Implantology. Stuttgart: Thieme Verlag, 1995, 91–124.

29. Wilson DJ. Ridge mapping for determination of alveolar ridge width. Int Oral Maxillofac Implants 1989(4): 41–46.

30. Marizola R, Derbabian K, Donovan T, and Arcidiacono A. The science of communicating the art of esthetic dentistry. Part I: Patient–dentist–patient communication. J Esthet Dent 2000(12): 131–138.

31. Roge M and Preston JD. Color, light, and perception of form. Quintessence Int 1987(18): 391–396.

32. Rifkin L and Materdomini D. Facial/lip reproduction system for anterior restorations. J Esthet Dent 1993(5): 126–131

33. Wood RE and Lee L. Systematic interpretation of pathologic conditions on oral radiographs. Ontario Dentist 1994(Jan/Feb): 17–22.

34. Gher ME and Richardson AC. The accuracy of dental radiographic techniques used for evaluation of implant fixture placement. Int J PeriodontRest Dent 1995(15): 268–283.

35. Garg AK and Vicari A. Radiographic modalities for diagnosis and treatment planning in implant dentistry. Implant Soc 1995(5): 7–11.

36. Farman AG and Farman TT. Radiovisiography-ui: A sensor to rival direct exposure intra-oral x-ray film. Int J Computerized Dent 1999 2(3): 183–196.

37. Reddy MS and Wang IC. Radiographic determinants of implant performance. Adv Dent Res 1999(13): 136–145.

38. James, RA, Lozada JL, and Truitt HP. Computer tomography (CT) applications in implant dentistry. J Oral Implantol 1991(17): 10–15.

39. Dula K, Mini R, Van der Stelt PF, and Buser D. The radiographic assessment of implant patients: Decision-making criteria. Int J Oral Maxillofac Implants 2001(16): 80–89.

40. Reddy MS, Mayfield-Donahoo T, Vanderven FJ, and Jeffcoat MK. A comparison of the diagnostic advantages of panoramic radiography and computed tomography scanning for placement of root form dental implants. Clin Oral Implant Res 1994(5): 229–238.

41. Potter BJ, Shrout MK, Russell CM, and Sharawy M. Implant site assessment using panoramic cross-sectional tomographic imaging. Oral Surg Oral Med Oral Pathol Oral Radiol Endod 1997(84): 436–442.

42. Scaf G, Lurie AG, Mosier KM, Kantor ML, Ramsby GR, and Freedman ML. Dosimetry and cost of imaging osseointegrated implants with film-based and computed tomography. Oral Surg Oral Med Oral Pathol Oral Radiol Endod 1997(83): 41–48.

43. Schartz MS, Rothman SL, Chavetz W, and Rhodes M. Computed tomography in dental implant surgery. Dent Clin North Am 1989(33): 565–597.

44. Zabalegui J, Gil JA, and Zabalegui B. Magnetic resonance imaging as an adjunctive diagnostic aid in patient selection for endosseous implants, preliminary study. Int J Oral Maxillofac Implants. 1990(5): 283–287.

45. Stein RS, Kuwata M.A. Dentist and a dental technologist analyze current ceramometal procedures. Dent Clin North Am 1977(21): 729–749.

46. Frush JP and Fisher RD. The dynesthetic interpretation of the dentogenic concept. J Prosthet Dent 1958(8): 558–581.

47. Meyenberg KH. Modified porcelain-fused-to-metal restorations and porcelain laminates for anterior aesthetics. Pract Periodont Aesthet Dent 1995 7(8): 33–44.

48. Palmquist S, and Swartz B. Artificial crowns and fixed partial dentures 18 to 23 years after placement. Int J Prosthodont 1993(6): 279–285.

49. Schwartz NL, Whitsett LD, Berry TG, and Stewart JL. Unserviceable crowns and fixed partial dentures: Lifespan and causes of loss of serviceability. J Am Dent Assoc 1970(81): 1395–1401.

50. Meyenberg KH and Imoberdorf MJ. The aesthetic challenges of single tooth replacement: A comparison of treatment alternatives. Pract Periodont Aesthet Dent 1997 9(7): 727–735.

51. Koth DL. Full crown restorations and gingival inflammation in a controlled population. J Prosthet Dent 1982(48): 681–685.

52. Silness J. Periodontal conditions in patients treated with dental bridges. The relationship between the location of the crown margin and the periodontal condition. J Periodontol Res 1970(5): 225–229.

53. Rochette AL. Attachment of a splint to enamel of lower anterior teeth. J Prosthet Dent 1986(56): 416–421.

54. Hussey DL, Pagni C, and Linden G L. Performance of 400 adhesive bridges fitted in a restorative dentistry department. J Dent 1991(19): 221–225.

55. Williams VD, Thayer KE, Denehy GE, and Boyer DB. Cast metal, resin bonded prosthesis: A 10-year retrospective study. J Prosthet Dent 1989(61): 436–441.

56. Hansson O. Clinical results with resin-bonded prostheses and an adhesive cement. Quintessence Int 1994(25): 125–132.

57. Barrack G and Bretz WA. A long term prospective study of the acid etched-cast restoration. Int J Prosthodont 1993(6): 428–434.

58. Priest GF. Failure rates of restorations for single-tooth replacement. Int J Prosthodont 1996(9): 38–45.

59. Haas R, Mensdorff-Pouilly N, Mailath G, and Watzek G. Brånemark single tooth implants: A preliminary report of 76 implants. J Prosthet Dent 1995(73): 274–279.

60. Jemt T, Lekholm U, and Grondahl K. Three-year follow-up study of early single implant restorations ad modum Branemark. Int J Periodont Rest Dent 1990(10): 340–349.

61. Schwarz MS. Mechanical complications of dental implants. Clin Oral Implant Res 2000 11(Suppl. 1): 156–158

62. Grunder U, Spielman H-P, and Gaberthuel T. Implant-supported single tooth replacement in the aesthetic region: A complex challenge. Pract Periodont Aesthet Dent 1996 8(9): 835–842.

63. Bloomberg S, and Linquist L. Psychological reactions to edentulousness and treatment with jawbone-anchored bridges. Acta Psychiatr Scand 1983(68): 251–262.

64. Tuominen R, Ranta K, and Paunio I. Wearing of removable partial dentures in relation to periodontal pockets. J Oral Rehab 1989(16): 119–126.

65. Wright PS, Hellyer PH, Beighton D, et al. Relationship of removable partial denture use to root caries in an older population. Int J Prosthodont 1992(5): 39–46.

66. Witter DJ, van Elteren P, Käyser AF, and van Rossum MJ. The effect of removable partial dentures on the oral function in shortened dental arches. J Oral Rehab 1989(16): 27–33.

67. Cowan RD, Gilbert JA, Elledge DA, and McGlynn FD. Patient use of removable partial dentures: Two- and four-year telephone interviews. J Prosthet Dent 1991(65): 668–670.

68. Budtz-Jøgensen E and Isidor F. Cantilever bridges or removable partial dentures in geriatric patients: A two-year study. J Oral Rehab 1987(14): 239–249.

69. Hebel K, Gajjar R, and Hofstede T. Single-tooth replacement: Bridge vs. implant supported restoration. J Can Dent Assoc 2000(66): 435–438.

70. Balshi TJ and Garver DG. Osseointegration: The efficacy of the transitional denture. Int J Oral Maxillofac Implants 1986(1): 113–118.

71. Biggs WF. Placement of a custom implant provisional restoration at the second-stage surgery for improved gingival management: A clinical report. J Prosthet Dent 1996(75): 231–233.

72. Soballe K, Hansen ES, Brockstedt-Rasmussen H, Pedersen CM, and Bunger C. Hydroxyapatite coating enhances fixation of porous coated implants. Acta Orthop Scand 1990 61(4): 299–306.

73. Lewis S, Parel S, and Faulkner R. Provisional implant-supported fixed restorations. Int J Oral Maxillofac Implants 1995(10): 319–325.

74. Brown MS, and Tarnow DP. Fixed provisionalization with transitional implants for partially edentulous patients: A case report. Pract Periodont Aesthet Dent 2001(13): 123–127.

75. Froum S, Ematiaz S, and Bloom MJ. The use of transitional implants for immediate fixed temporary prosthesis in cases of implant restorations. Pract Periodont Aesthet Dent 1997(10): 737.

76. Berglundh T, and Lindhe J. Dimension of the peri-implant mucosa: Biological width revisited. J Clin Periodontol 1996(23): 971–973.

77. Tarnow DP and Eskow RN. Preservation of implant esthetics: Soft and restorative considerations. J Esthet Dent 1995(8): 12–19.

78. Seibert JS and Salama H. Alveolar ridge preservation and reconstruction. Periodontol 2000 1996(6): 69–84.

79. Adell R, Eriksson B, Lekholm U, et al. Long-term follow-up study of osseointegrated implants in the treatment of totally edentulous jaws. Int J Oral Maxillofac Implants 1990(5): 347–359.

80. Adell R Lekholm U, Rockler B, and Brånemark PI. A 15-year study of osseointegrated implants in the treatment of the edentulous jaw. Int J Oral Surg 1981(10): 387–416.

81. Cox JF and Zarb GA. The longitudinal clinical efficacy of osseointegrated dental implants: A 3-year report. Int J Oral Maxillofac Implants 1987(2): 91–100.

82. Zarb GA and Schmitt A. the longitudinal clinical effectiveness of osseointegrated dental implants: The Toronto study. Part III: Problems and complications encountered. J Prosthet Dent 1990(64): 185–194.

83. Lang NP and Löe H. The relationship between the width of keratinized gingiva and gingival health. J Periodontol 1972(43): 623–627.

84. Dorfman HS, Kennedy JE, and Bird WC. Longitudinal evaluation of free autogenous gingival autografts. J Clin Periodontol 1980(7): 316–324.

85. Stetler KJ and Bissada NF. Significance of the width of keratinized gingiva on the periodontal status of teeth with submarginal restorations. J Periodontol 1987(58): 696–700.

86. Bengazi F, Wennstrom L, and Lekholm U. Recession of the soft tissue margin at oral implants: A 2-year longitudinal prospective study. Clin Oral Implant Res 1996(7): 303–310.

87. Glickman I. Clinical Periodontology, 4th ed. Philadelphia: W. B. Saunders, 1972.

88. Ochsenbein C and Ross S. A concept of osseous surgery and its clinical applications. In Ward HL and Chas C, eds. A Periodontal Point of View. Springfield, IL: Charles C. Thomas, 1973.

89. Weisgold A. Contours of the full crown restoration. Alpha Omegan 1977(10): 77–89.

90. Olsson M and Lindhe J. Periodontal characteristics in individuals with varying forms of the upper central incisors. J Clin Periodontol 1991(18): 78–82.

91. Gargiulo AW, Wentz FM, and Orban B. Dimensions and relations of the dentogingival junction in humans. J Periodontol 1961(32): 261–267.

92. Jansen, CE and Weisgold A. Presurgical treatment planning for the anterior single-tooth implant restoration. Compend Cont Educ Dent 1995(16): 746–762.

93. Esposito M, Ekestubbe A, and Gröndahl K. Radiological evaluation of marginal bone loss at tooth surfaces facing single Brånemark implants. Clin Oral Implant Res 1993(4): 151–157.

94. Tarnow D, Magner A, and Fletcher P. The effect of the distance from the contact point to the crest of bone on the presence or absence of the interproximal papilla. J Periodontol 1992(63): 995–996.

95. Misch CE. Divisions of available bone. In Misch CE, ed. Contemporary Implant Dentistry. St. Louis: Mosby, 1999, 89–108.

96. Friberg B, Sennerby L, Roos J, and Lekholm U. Identification of bone quality in conjunction with insertion of titanium implants. A pilot study in jaw autopsy specimens. Clin Oral Implant Res 1995(4): 213.

97. Holmes DC and Loftus JT. Influence of bone quality on stress distribution for endosseous implants. J Oral Implantol 1997(23): 104.

98. Lam RV. Contour changes of the alveolar process following extraction. J Prosthet Dent 1967(17): 21–27.

99. Parkinson CF. Similarities in resorption patterns of maxillary and mandibular ridges. J Prosthet Dent 1978(39): 598–602.

100. Pietrokovski J, Sorin S, and Hirschfeld Z. The residual ridge in partially edentulous patients. J Prosthet Dent 1967(36): 150–157.

101. Tallgren A. The continuing reduction of the residual alveolar ridges in complete denture wearers. A mixed longitudinal study covering 25 years. J Prosthet Dent 1972(27): 120–132.

102. Salama H and Salama M. The role of orthodontic extrusive remodeling in the enhancement of soft and hard tissue profiles prior to implant placement: A systematic approach to the management of extraction site defects. Int J Periodont Rest Dent 1993(13): 313–333.

103. Misch EC. Bone density: A key Determinant for clinical success. In Misch CE, ed. Contemporary Implant Dentistry, St. Louis: Mosby, 1999, 109–118.

104. Pietrokowki J. The bony residual ridge in man. J Prosthet Dent 1975(34): 456–462.

105. Zaher A, personal communication, Alexandria, Egypt, 2000.

106. Salama H, Salama M, and Kelly J. The orthodontic-periodontal connection in implant site development. Pract Periodont Aesthet Dent 1996(8): 923–932.

107. Ingber JS. Forced eruption, Part I. A method of treating isolated one and two wall infrabony defects—Rationale and case report. J Periodontol 1974 45(4): 199–206

108. Brown IS. The effect of orthodontic therapy on certain types of periodontal defects. J Periodontol 1973 44(12): 742–756

109. Bruskin R, Castellon P, and Hochstedler J. Orthodontic extrusion and orthodontic extraction in preprosthetic treatment using implant therapy. Pract Periodont Aesthet Dent 2000(12): 213–221.

110. Beitan K. Clinical and histological observations on tooth movement during and after orthodontic treatment. Am J Orthod 1967(53): 721–745.

111. Potashnick SR and Rosenberg ES. Forced eruption: Principles in periodontics and restorative dentistry. J Prosthet Dent 1982(48): 141–148.

112. Meyer MD and Bruce DM. Implant site development using orthodontic extrusion: A case report. N Z Dent J 2000(96): 18–20.

113. El Askary AS, Meffert RM, and Griffin T. Why do dental implants fail? Part I. Implant Dent 1999(8): 173–185.

114. Sussman HI, and Moss SS. Localized osteomyelitis secondary to endodontic-implant pathosis: A case report. J Periodontol 1993(64): 306–310.

115. Sussman HI. Endodontic pathology leading to implant failure: A case report. J Oral Implantol 1997(23): 112–115.

116. Novaes AB, Jr., and Novaes AB. Immediate implants placed into infected sites: A clinical report. Int J Oral Maxillofac Implants 1995(10): 609–613.

117. A Ameed, Personal communications, London, United Kingdom, 2001.

118. Hulsey CM. An esthetic evaluation of lip-teeth relationships present in the smile. Am J Orthod 1970(57): 132–144.

119. Burstone CJ. Lip posture and its significance in treatment planning. Am J Orthod 1967(53): 262–284.

120. Weickersheimer PB. Steiner analysis. In Jacobson A, ed. Radiographic Cephalometry. Carol Stream, IL: Quintessence Publishing, 1995, 83–85.

121. Viazis AD. A new measurement of profile esthetics. J Clin Orthod 1991(25): 15–20.

122. Rifkin R. Facial analysis: A comprehensive approach to treatment planning in aesthetic dentistry. Pract Periodont Aesthet Dent 2000(12): 865–871.

123. Martone AL and Edwards LF. Anatomy of the mouth and related structures. Part 1. The face. J Prosthet Dent 1978(39): 128–134.

124. Maritato FR and Douglas JR. A positive guide to anterior tooth placement. J Prosthet Dent 1964(14): 848.

125. Philips ED. The anatomy of a smile. Oral Health 1996(86): 7–9, 11–13.

126. Kent G. Effect of osseointegrated implants on psychological and social well-being: A literature review. J Prosthet Dent 1992(68): 515–518.

127. Tjan AHL and Miller GD. Some esthetic factors in smile. J Prosthet Dent 1984;51: 24–28; Hulsey CM. An esthetic evaluation of lip-teeth relationships present in the smile. Am J Orthod 1970(57): 132–144.

128. Philips ED. The classifications of smile patterns. J Can Dent Assoc 1999 65(May): 252–254.

129. Rubin LR. The anatomy of a smile: Its importance in the treatment of facial paralysis. Plast Reconstr Surg 1974(53): 384–387.

130. Morley J. Smile design—Specific consideration. J Calif Dent Assoc 1997(25): 633–637.

131. Golub-Evans J. Unity and variety: Essential ingredients of a smile design. Curr Opin Cosmet Dent 1994:1–5.

132. Lorobardi RE.The principles of visual perception and their clinical application to denture esthetics. J Prosthet Dent 1973(29): 1973

133. Frush JP and Fisher RD. How dentogenic restorations interpret the sex factor. J Prosthet Dent 1956(6): 160–172.

134. Golub J. Male/female standards blend esthetic styles. Dent Mag 1988(25): 25.

135. Allen EP. Use of Mucogingival surgical procedures to enhance esthetics. Dent Clin North Am 1988(32): 307–330.

136. W. Dickerson, Trilogy of creating on esthetic smile, Tech Update 1(1996): 1–7.

137. Moskowitz M and Nayyar A. Determinants of dental esthetics: A rational for smile analysis and treatment. Compend Cont Educ Dent 1995(16): 1164–1186.

138. Rufenacht C. Fundamentals of Esthetics. Carol Stream, IL: Quintessence, 1990, 77–126.

139. Perel M. Achieving critical emergence profile for the anterior tooth implant. Dent Implantol Update 1993(4): 88–92.

140. Croll BM. Emergence profiles in natural tooth contour. Part I: Photographic observations. J Prosthet Dent 1989(62): 374–379.

141. Touati B. The double guidance concept. Pract Periodont Aesthet Dent 1997(9): 1089–1094.

142. Weisgold AS, Arnoux JP, and Lu J. Single-tooth anterior implant: A word of caution. J Esthet Dent 1997(9): 225–233.

143. Arlin ML. Optimal placement of osseointegrated implants. J Can Dent Assoc 1990(56): 873–876.

144. Garber DA. The esthetic dental implant: Letting the restoration be the guide. J Am Dent Assoc 1995(126): 319–325.

145. Palacci P. Optimal implant positioning. In Palacci P and Erecsson I. Esthetic Implant Dentistry. Soft and Hard Tissue Management. Berlin: Quintessence, 2001, 101–135.

146. Cowan PW. Surgical templates for the placement of osseointegrated implants. Quintessence Int 1990(2): 391–396.

147. Touati B. The double guidance concept. Int J Dent Symp 1997(4): 4–9.

148. Tarnow DP and Eskow RN. Considerations for single unit esthetic implant restorations. Compend Cont Educ Dent 1995(16): 778–788.

149. Engelman MJ, Sorensen JA, and Moy P. Optimum placement of osseointegrated implants. J Prosthet Dent 1988(59): 467–473.

150. Shepherd NJ. A general dentist's guide to proper implant placement from an oral surgeon's perspective. Compend Cont Educ Dent 1996(27): 118–130.

151. Kennedy BD, Collins TA, and Kline, PC. Simplified guide for precise implant placement: A technical note. Int J Oral Maxillofac Implants 1998(13): 684–688.

152. Becker CM and Kaiser DA. Surgical guide for dental implant placement. J Prosthet Dent 2000(83): 248–251.

153. Cenrell MC and Sahin S. Fabrication of a dual-purpose surgical template for correct labiopalatal positioning of dental implants. Int J Oral Maxillofac Implants 2000(15): 278–282.

154. Verdi MA and Morgano SM. A dual-purpose stent for the implant-supported prosthesis. J Prosthet Dent 1993(69): 276–280.

155. Klein M and Abrams M. Computer-guided surgery utilizing a computer-milled surgical template, Pract Proced Aesthet Dent 2001(13): 165–169.

156. Minoretti R, Merz BR, and Triaca A. Predetermined implant positioning by means of a Novel guide template technique. Clin Oral Implant Res 2000(11): 266–272.

157. Tarnow D and Fletcher P. The two to three months post-extraction placement of root form implants: A useful compromise. Implants. Clin Rev Dent 1993(2): 1–8.

158. Laney WR. Selecting edentulous patients for tissue-integrated prosthesis. Int J Oral Maxillofac Implants 1986(1): 129–138.

159. Atwood DA and Coy DA. Clinical, cephalometric and densitometric study of reduction of residual ridge. J Prosthet Dent 1971(26): 280–293.

160. Johnson K. A study of the dimensional changes occurring in the maxilla after tooth extraction. Part I: Normal healing. Aust Dent J 1963(8): 428–433.

161. Carlsson GE, Bergman B, and Headegard B. Changes in contour of the maxillary alveolar process under immediate dentures. A longitudinal clinical and x-ray cephalometric study covering 5 years. Acta Odontol Scand 1967(25): 45–75.

162. Brazilay I et al. Immediate implantation of pure titanium threaded implants into extraction sockets. J Dent Res 1988(67): 234.

163. Becker W and Becker BE. Guided tissue regeneration for implants placed into extraction sockets and for implant dehiscences: Surgical techniques and case reports. Int J Periodont Rest Dent 1990(10): 377–391.

164. Lazzara RJ. Immediate implant placement into extraction sites: Surgical and restorative advantages. Int J Periodont Rest Dent 1989(9): 333–343.

165. Dennisen HW, Kalk W, Veldhuis HAH, and Van Waas MAJ. Anatomic consideration for preventive implantation. Int J Oral Maxillofac Implants 1993(8): 191–196.

166. Sclar AG. Ridge preservation for optimum esthetics and function: The "Bio-Col" technique. Postgrad Dent 1999(6): 3–11.

167. Mensdorff-Pouilly N, Haas R, Mailath G, and Watzek G. The immediate implant: A retrospective study comparing the different types of immediate implantation. Int J Oral Maxillofac Implants 1994(9): 571–578.

168. Watzek G, Haider R, Mensdorff-Pouilly N, and Haas R. Immediate and delayed implantation for complete restoration of the jaw following extraction of all residual teeth: A retrospective study comparing different types of serial immediate implantation. Int J Oral Maxillofac Implants 1995(10): 561–567.

169. Rosenquist B and Grenthe B. Immediate placement of implants into extraction sockets: Implant survival, Int J Oral Maxillofac Implants 1996(11): 205–209.

170. Small PN, Tarnow DP, and Cho SC. Gingival recession around standard-diameter implants: A 3- to 5-year longitudinal prospective study. Pract Proced Aesthet Dent 2001(13): 143–146.

171. Gelb DA. Immediate implant surgery: Three-year retro-spective evaluation of 50 consecutive cases. Int J Oral Maxillofac Implants. 1993(8): 388–399.

172. Ashman A, LoPoint J, and Rosenlicht J. Ridge augmentation for immediate post-extraction implants: Eight-year retrospective study. Pract Periodont Aesthet Dent 1995(7): 85–95.

173. Garber DA and Belser UC. Restoration-drive implant placement with restoration-generated site development. Compend Contin Educ Dent 1995(16): 796–804.

174. Meltzer A. Non-resorbable membrane-assisted bone regeneration: Stabilization and the avoidance of micro-movement. Dent Implantol Update1995(6): 45–48.

175. Tehemar SH. Classification and treatment modalities for immediate implantation. Part I: Hard and soft tissue status. Implant Dent 1999(8): 54–60.

176. Saadoun AP and La Gall M. Periodontal implications in implant treatment planning for aesthetic results. Pract Periodont Aesthet Dent 1998(11): 655–664.

177. Wheeler SL, Vogel RE, and Casellini R. Tissue preservation and maintenance of optimum esthetics: A clinical report. Int J Oral Maxillofac Implants 2000(15): 265–271.

178. Ogiso M, Tabata T, Ramonito R, and Borgese D. Delay method of implantation enhances implant-bone binding: A comparison with the conventional method. Oral Maxillofac Implants 1995(10): 415–420.

179. Misch CE, Misch FD, and Misch CM. A modified socket seal surgery with composite graft approach. J Oral Implantol 1999(4): 244–250.

180. Buser D, Mericske-Stern R, Bernard JP, Behneke A, Behneke N, Hirt HP, Belser UC, and Lang NP. Long-term evaluation of non-submerged ITI implants. Part 1: Eight-year life table analysis of a prospective multicenter study with 2359 implants. Clin Oral Implant Res 1997(8): 161–172.

181. Buser D, Mericske-Stern R, Dula K, and Lang NP. Clinical experience with one-stage, non-submerged dental implants. Adv Dent Res 1999(13): 153–161.

182. Cornelini R, Scarano A, Covani U, Petrone G, and Piattelli A. Immediate one-stage postextraction implant: A human clinical and histologic case report. Int J Oral Maxillofac Implants 2000(15): 432–437.

183. Misch C.E. Single tooth implant. In Misch CE, ed. Contemporary Implant Dentistry. St. Louis: Mosby, 1999, 397–428.

El Askary-Meffert Failure Checklist

PERSONAL DATA:

Name: ....
Age: ....   Sex: ....
Date of Examination: ....
Name of Examiner: ....
Functioning Lifetime of the Implant: ....

EXAMINATION:

| **1. Failure Reason:** |
| Host (Physical or Psychological) |
| Surgical Placement |
| Implant Selection |
| Restorative |

| **2. Failure Timing:** |
| Before Stage II (Post Surgery) |
| At Stage II (with healing head and/or abutment insertion) |
| Post Restorative |

| **3. Failure Condition:** |
| Surviving |
| Ailing |
| Failing |
| Failed |

| **4. Responsible Personnel:** |
| General Dentist |
| Surgeon |
| Prosthodontist |
| Periodontist |
| Hygienist |
| Lab. Technician |
| Patient |

| **5. Failure Mode:** |
| Lack of Osseointegration (usually mobility) |
| Unacceptable Esthetics |
| Functional Problems |
| Psychological Problems |

| **6. Failure According to Tissue Type:** |
| Soft Tissue Problems (inc. Lack of keratinized tissue, inflammation, etc.) |
| Bone Loss (inc. Radiographic changes, etc.) |
| Soft and Hard Tissue Changes |

| **7. Failure According to Origin:** |
| Peri-implantitis (infective process, bacterial origin) |
| Retrograde peri-implantitis (traumatic occlusion origin, non-infective, forces "off long-axis", premature or excessive loading) |

REMARKS:
(Please elaborate on the failure cause e.g. HOST ➝ due to systemic conditions e.g. Diabetes mellitus)
....
....
....
....
....

signed

FIGURE 3.2. El Askary-Meffert failure checklist, showing that an unacceptable aesthetic result with dental implants is considered a failed condition.

The unique human periodontium is divided into two basic biotypes: the thin scalloped biotype and the thick flat biotype.[21–23] Each biotype has its own particular tooth anatomy and osseous topography.[24,25]

Thin scalloped tissue biotype is characterized by narrow, tapered roots and a triangular or cylindrical crown shape; the contact areas are located more incisally with a reduced cervical convexity. Therefore the interproximal papillae are located in an incisal position and do not totally fill the whole embrasure space, which explains their designation as "scalloped." Due to the relatively small diameter and tapered form of the roots of the thin scalloped biotype, the interradicular bone is wider than in the thick flat biotype.[26–28]

The thick flat biotype is characterized by a bulbous root form and a square crown shape. In some areas the wide root diameter in this biotype can have the same width as the widest part of the crown. Wide contact areas are located more apically, and eventually the interproximal papillae fill all of the embrasure space.

Based on the foregoing, when a missing single tooth with thin scalloped tissue biotype is to be restored with a dental implant, the final aesthetic result might not be entirely predictable, because recession of the interproximal papilla and its surrounding gingival structures might be a likely event. This is due to the reduced amount of keratinized tissues and the fragile nature of the soft tissue that characterizes this biotype. Also, the greater vertical distance of undulation between the edge of the implant's cervix and the interproximal bone margin stimulates mild bone resorption, which leads to unsymmetrical peri-implant tissue margins when compared with the contralateral side.[29] Any additional osseous remodeling will result in further shortening of the already short papillae, thus complicating aesthetics.[30]

On the other hand, when a dental implant is placed in the thick tissue biotype, the vertical undulation space located between the edge of the implant's cervix and the margin of the interproximal bone is minimized. This will not be of any serious significant clinical concern.[29] The thick flat tissue biotype certainly offers more predictable aesthetic treatment outcome than the thin scalloped biotype. Therefore, patients with the thick flat biotype are generally considered more favorable candidates for achieving and maintaining acceptable aesthetic results with implant placement and restorative therapy. That being the case, recognition and assessment of the tissue biotype before commencing implant therapy is important. The proper assessment of the tissue biotype preoperatively will mandate a specific surgical approach that suits each type. For example, in the thin scalloped tissue biotype, it seemed that a flapless approach to implant placement can reduce the tendency for postoperative soft tissue shrinkage and healing complications.

AESTHETIC IMPLANT DESIGN

The newly designed dental implants offer several modifications compared with the old classic ones; the changes involve new implant surface treatments, new interface connections, versatile sizes, and new implant-related prosthetic components. This has led to increased awareness of the clinicians to challenge the clinical outcome of dental implants and to take dental implants to a new horizon. The newly introduced dental implant designs have led the clinicians to dramatically improve the clinical outcome of dental implants from the aesthetic standpoint and to take implant-supported restorations to new levels. Thus, selection of the optimum implant design and size is now becoming an integral part of every treatment plan that seeks a superior aesthetic outcome.

The implants of choice that are available to restore missing teeth are either endosseous screws or cylinders. The standard screw-type body is 3.75 mm in diameter, and the diameter of its platform flares up to 4.1 mm.[31] The cylinder design of endosseous implants usually has a 4-mm body diameter and the same platform dimensions as the screw type.[6]

The abutments for the cylindrical and screw type implants start with the same diameter as the implant's platform and then flare out to 4.5 or 5 mm. While these dimensions might vary somewhat among implant manufacturers or due to laboratory modifications of the abutment, generally most of the standard implant diameters will require a crown with a diameter of a minimum of 5.5 mm at the CEJ level and 7 mm at the level of the contact points when a missing central incisor is being restored,[29] for instance. In order to obtain natural biological contours of implant supported restorations, the difference in the diameter of the implant and the cervical dimension of the missing tooth should be compensated for. This is accomplished either by tissue expansion procedures through the provisional prosthesis to allow a smooth transition from the implant head diameter to that of the natural tooth or by using wide implants with abutments that have a diameter approximately similar to that of missing tooth. Selecting implant diameter that is wider than the tooth to be replaced will result in a crown that is incorrect in its size and does not biologically fit with the surrounding tissues (Fig. 3.3). In conclusion, the use of a wide implant diameter that exceeds the natural biological dimensions will jeopardize not only aesthetics but also function. The implant diameter is directly related to the root diameter at the crest of the alveolar ridge. For example, if a missing maxillary central incisor to be replaced with a dental implant has a diameter that ranges between 7 and 8.5 mm at the CEJ level and between 5 and 6 mm at the bone level, the diameter of the implant to be used may vary from 4 to 6 mm, and so forth.[26] Therefore the diameter of the implant should be related to the diameter of the root at the bone emergence level and not the CEJ level, because if the diameter of the implant exceeds the diameter of the root at the bone level, this will eventually cause crestal bone resorption. The diameter of the missing tooth can be verified by measuring the dimensions of the same tooth on the contralateral side, or by studying an old study cast or photograph for the

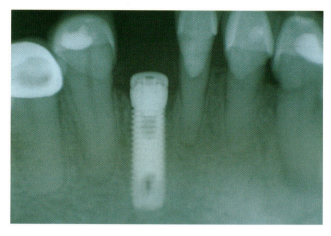

FIGURE 3.3. An implant replacing the mandibular lateral incisor is wider than the original missing tooth dimension at the crestal bone level; this leads to a bulky restoration at the emergence level compared with its adjacent natural tooth.

patient. The width of the implant dictates its position in the alveolar ridge; wider implants are less apically positioned while narrow diameter implants are more apically placed in order to allow for "running room" to stack the prosthetic components in.

It is noteworthy that any attempt to follow a specific formula for selecting a particular implant diameter for a specific tooth will be very unsatisfactory, because there are many other variables that must be considered in the implant diameter selection process. Some of these include variations in the tissue biotype, differences in the size of the same tooth's diameter among different individuals, changes that occur to the remaining bone after extraction, the altered soft tissue contours, and the variation in implant diameters. Thus, the clinician's personal evaluation will be the best tool for selecting the proper implant size. Adhering to specific ready-made charts may not work well in many clinical conditions and can sometimes lead to confusion.

AESTHETIC IMPLANT POSITIONING

Accurate implant positioning enhances natural aesthetics; an implant should not be inserted into the alveolar ridge at random wherever there is a space available because the implant requires sufficient osseous dimensions and restorative dimensions. These dimensions are not always related to one another, and sometimes one dimension may be adequate while the other is not; the balance between these two dimensions will lead to the

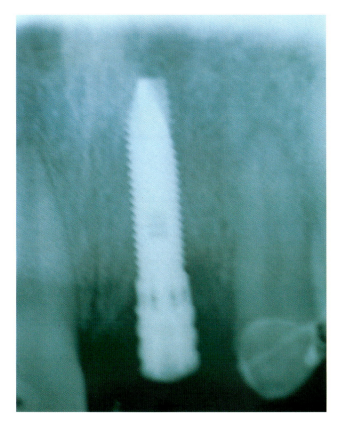

FIGURE 3.4a. Optimal mesiodistal positioning of an implant.

optimal implant positioning.[6] Certain guidelines are presented to assist in placing the implant in a three-dimensional fashion; the three dimensions are related to the lateral axis (mesiodistal dimension), the sagittal axis (labiopalatal dimension), and the coronal axis (apicoincisal dimension).

MESIODISTAL POSITIONING

The mesiodistal position of the implant in relation to the adjacent teeth has a direct impact on the aesthetic outcome and the integrity of the future restoration contours. It also directly affects postoperative hygiene maintenance around dental implants. In ideal soft and hard tissue conditions, the implant should be positioned midway in the center of the mesiodistal space in order to obtain a centralized restoration if a missing single tooth is being restored (Fig. 3.4a). Care should be exercised to avoid placing the implant in a position too close to the interdental papilla (Fig. 3.4b). Failure to heed this precaution can induce pressure on the papillary soft tissue that hinders hygiene measures and potentially jeopardizes aesthetics (Fig. 3.5). Improper mesiodistal positioning may

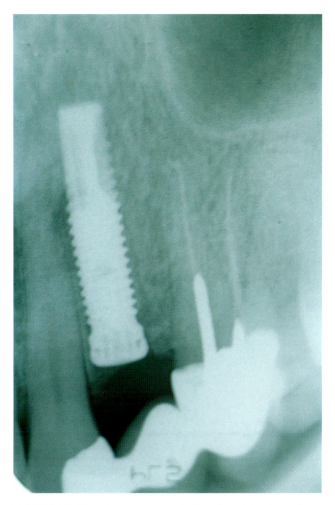

FIGURE 3.4b. Improper mesiodistal positioning of an implant.

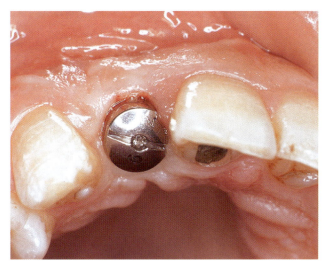

FIGURE 3.5. Healing abutment in place, exerting pressure on the interdental papilla due to the improper mesiodistal placement of the implant body.

also affect the periodontium of the adjacent tooth to the implant site; it can compromise the blood supply, thus leading to possible external root resorption.[32] This last-mentioned complication might underscore the importance of using cylindrical root form dental implants. The use of tapered implant design may reduce the chance of adjacent root approximation (Fig. 3.6).

The presence of diastemas demands more careful mesiodistal positioning of dental implants. Here, the available mesiodistal space will be greater in width than the required space for the definitive restoration (Fig. 3.7). In such cases, the fabrication of a precise surgical template is valuable to ensure optimal implant positioning.[33] The misplacement of the implant in the space where diastema exists may cause irreversible aesthetic problems.

For single-tooth replacements, the formula for calculating the minimum space required for mesiodistal positioning of the implant should include the width of the periodontal ligament (average 0.25 mm) and a 1 mm

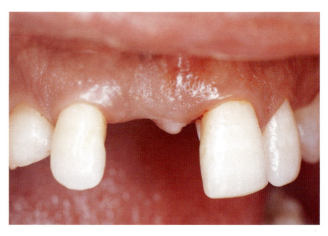

FIGURE 3.7.   Preoperative view of a missing left maxillary central incisor with preexisting median diastema that mandates accurate mesiodistal positioning of the implant.

zone of sound bone between the implant and the periodontal ligament of the adjacent natural tooth.[34] It must be remembered that the measurements accounting for the periodontal ligament and sound bone should be doubled to calculate both the mesial and distal aspects of the implant. Simply stated, the required distance for placing a 4 mm diameter implant between two teeth would be calculated by adding 1 mm + 0.25 mm + 4 mm + 0.25 mm + 1 mm. The resultant sum of 6.5 mm is the minimal space needed to position the implant mesiodistally. When multiple implants are used, the previous equation may be used by adding a distance of 2 or 3 mm between each implant.[35] However, these measurements are only recommended as a guideline, since every case should be approached on an individual basis. The mesiodistal position of an implant depends on the mesiodistal dimension of the edentulous space, the presence or absence of diastemas, and the adjacent root proximity.

LABIOPALATAL POSITIONING

The labiopalatal orientation of the implant directly influences the emergence profile of the final restoration. In order to ensure an implant-supported restoration with a flat emergence profile (Fig. 3.8), it is necessary to leave 1 mm of intact labial bone covering the implant surface (Fig. 3.9).[32] In perfect bone situations, the implant should be placed as close to the buccal contour as the volume of the available bone permits, rather than being centered along the residual ridge (Fig. 3.10).[5] Therefore, 6 mm of bone width is necessary to place a 4 mm diameter implant labiopalatally; this will leave a minimum amount of bone surrounding the implant fixture to keep it

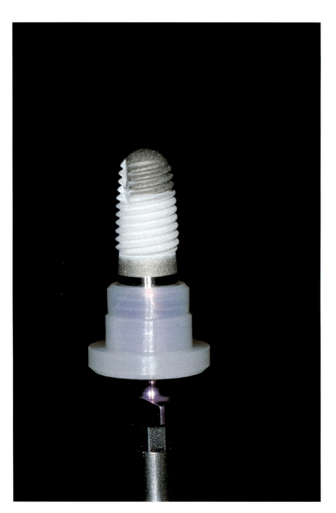

FIGURE 3.6.   Paragon tapered screw vent implant, 4.7 mm (Centerpulse, Dental Division, Carlsbad, California).

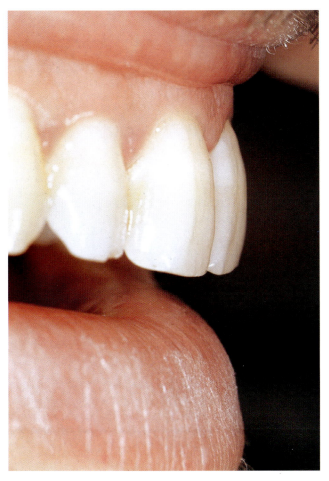

FIGURE 3.8.   Side view of maxillary teeth showing the natural flat emergence profile.

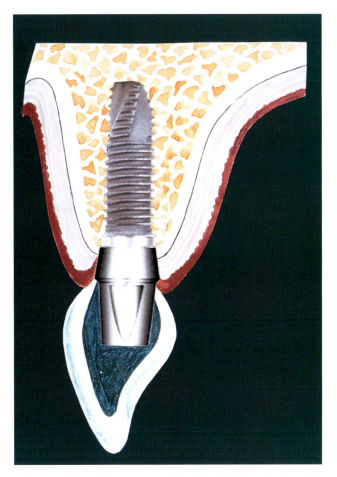

FIGURE 3.9.   Illustration of the ideal labiopalatal positioning of the implant fixture.

healthy. If the labiopalatal dimension is less than 6 mm, a small diameter implant may be used; if a large diameter implant is to be used, the bone dimension will need to be increased accordingly.[6]

If the implant is placed too far labially, it will violate the integrity of the labial plate of bone, leading to a final implant-supported restoration possessing bulky, overcontoured margins (Fig. 3.11a–c). This situation is clinically impossible to correct, even with the use of angulated abutments. In fact, angulated abutments might further complicate the situation, as their metallic gingival collar can potentially displace the soft tissue in a more labial direction, resulting in soft tissue recession or grayish, discolored gingiva.

Placement of the implant too far palatally will result in an increased distance between the labial edge of the implant and the highest point of the future crown contour at the emergence level (Fig. 3.12a–c). In other words, the final restoration will appear to be severely "ditched-in" when viewed sagittally. Consequently, fabrication of

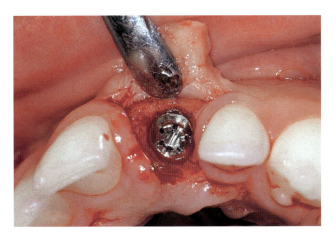

FIGURE 3.10.   The ideal labiopalatal placement of an implant fixture restoring a missing right maxillary central incisor clinically; note the remaining labial bone in relation to the fixture position.

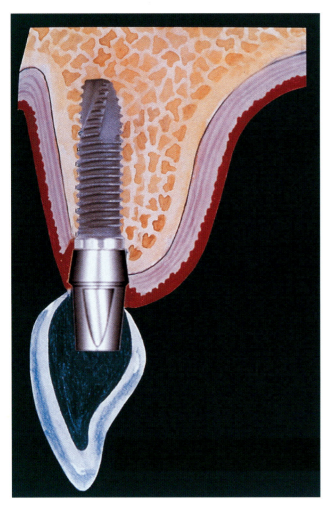

FIGURE 3.11a. An illustration showing too far labial placement of the implant fixture.

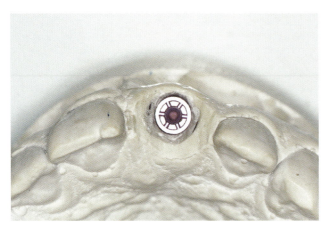

FIGURE 3.11b. A view showing a too far labially placed implant fixture on the study cast. Note the difference between the position of the natural tooth and the implant fixture.

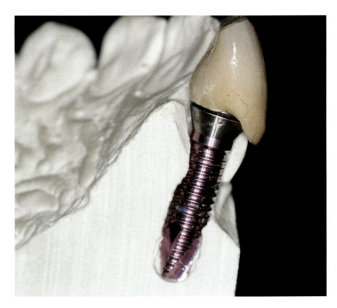

FIGURE 3.11c. A sagittal section of a study cast showing an implant fixture that is placed too far labially; note the violation of the labial plate of bone.

a restoration with a ridge-lap design at its labial margin to be aligned with the adjacent natural teeth is necessary. A ridge-lap design will hinder hygiene maintenance around the restoration labial contour, thereby facilitating plaque accumulation and leading to possible inflammation and apical migration of the gingival margin. This may be a potential threat to the implant's very existence, as pocket formation may ensue, resulting in implant failure. As a result of the modified ridge-lap design, there will be an increased strain on the implant surface due to an off-axis loading (Fig. 3.13a,b).[36]

Positioning the implant in relation to the sagittal axis within the labiopalatal dimension influences the implant angulation in the alveolar ridge as well. Some authors classify labiopalatal implant angulation in terms of its relation to the occlusal plane.[37] The implant may be inserted perpendicular to the occlusal plane, which provides a far more palatal positioning of the final restoration, resulting in a ridge-lap design of the restoration (Fig. 3.14a). An angulation of approximately 65 degrees, or 45 degrees to the occlusal plane, results in the most labial positioning of the implant head with optimal aesthetic results; this placement often requires using an angulated abutment (Fig. 3.14b).

The type of final abutment to be used somehow governs the labiopalatal positioning of the implant as well as its angulation. The final abutment and the final restoration should be determined before starting implant placement. There are two main types of final abutments, screw-retained abutments and cement-retained abut-

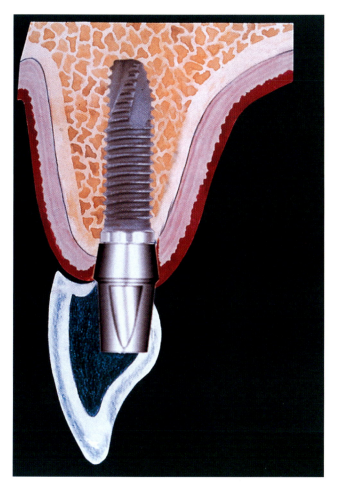

FIGURE 3.12a. An illustration showing too far palatal placement of an implant fixture.

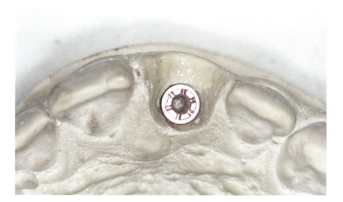

FIGURE 3.12b. Too far palatally placed implant fixture on the study cast; note the distance between the implant fixture to the labial plate of bone.

ments. The choice of positioning the implant fixture will depend on the space needed to gain accessibility to the abutment. For example, when cement-retained abut-

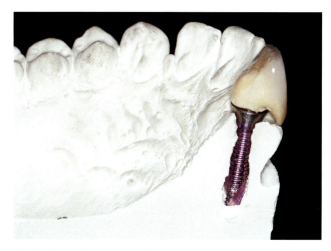

FIGURE 3.12c. A modified ridge-lap design of the crown to compensate for the too far palatal placement of the implant.

ments are used, the implant is positioned exactly in the center of the long axis of the future implant-supported crown (Fig. 3.15). On the other hand, when screw-retained abutments are used, the implant should be placed slightly palatal to the long axis of the crown, in order to access the connecting screw from the palatal side (Fig. 3.16).[38]

APICOINCISAL POSITIONING

One of the most critical areas in implant-supported restorations is the cervical region. Here lies the breaking point between an ordinary implant-supported restoration and an aesthetically superior implant-supported restoration; the latter is what demands skill and experience. The emergence profile and functional/mechanical requirements of the restorative components dictate the correct apicoincisal orientation of the implant to a great exent.[6] Apicoincisal positioning is no less important than the mesiodistal and labiopalatal positioning aspects of the implant, as this dimension determines the amount of exposure the final restoration will receive. This exposure dramatically affects the aesthetic outcome of the restoration.

Apicoincisal positioning of the implant allows the contours of the restoration to be developed in a progressive manner within the gingival sulcus so that the final restoration will appear to emerge naturally through the marginal gingival tissues (Fig. 3.17).[39] To create an implant-supported restoration that is successful from both the aesthetic and functional standpoints, several considerations must be weighed. These include the location and amount of space available for restoration, the topography of remaining bone, and the size and type of

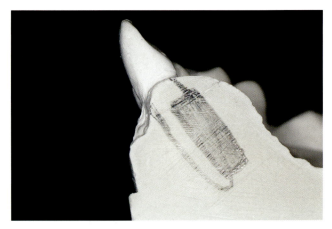

FIGURE 3.14a. Perpendicular placement of the implant to the occlusal plane that mandates slight palatal positioning.

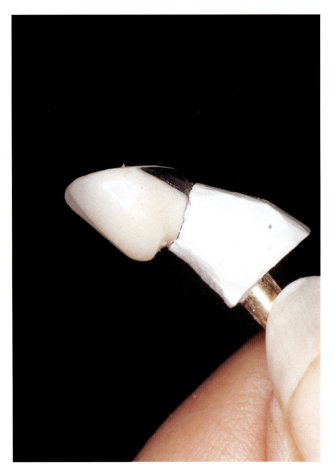

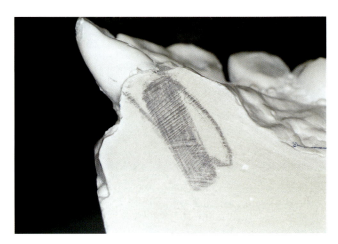

FIGURE 3.13a. Final restoration with a ridge-lap design to overcome palatally placed implant fixture.

FIGURE 3.14b. Implant angulation of 65 degrees that provides optimal aesthetic results.

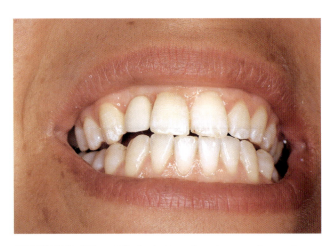

FIGURE 3.13b. Clinical view showing unpleasant aesthetic final result of an implant-supported crown (restoring upper right missing lateral incisor) due to the too far palatal placement of the implant fixture.

implant to be chosen. When multiple implants are to be used, a greater urgency for restoring gingival tissues sur-

rounding the new restorations exists. These implants should be placed at the alveolar crest within the circumference of the CEJ of the missing teeth to be restored. This will enable the clinician to develop appropriate embrasures on both sides adjoining the restorations as well as to develop the emergence profile.[5]

A difference exists between the fixture morphology and that of the natural tooth at the cervical level. Therefore, a transition from the narrow circular implant neck form to the natural tooth form is required. The ideal apicoincisal implant positioning will place the implant head 2–3 mm below a line connecting the gingival zeniths of the adjacent teeth. "Running room" should be allowed throughout the biological width of the implant when it is correctly positioned in an apicoincisal plane.[36] This "running room" is a space or leeway that lies 2–3 mm

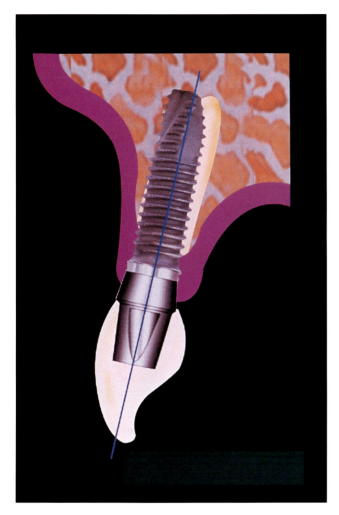

FIGURE 3.15. Illustration showing the long-axis positioning of the implant fixture in case of using a cement-retained abutment.

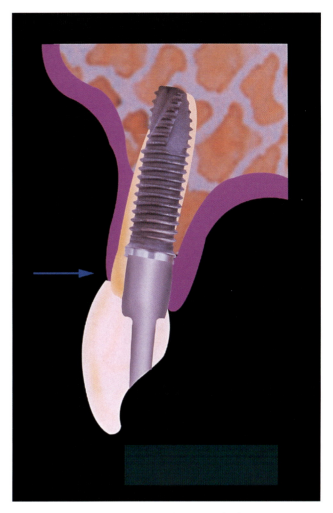

FIGURE 3.16. Illustration showing the long-axis positioning of the implant in case of using a screw-retained abutment.

apical to an imaginary line connecting the gingival zeniths of the neighboring dentition (Fig. 3.18). This room allows for stacking and building up of prosthetic components to create the natural contours of the final restoration. The use of anatomical abutments to provide the same cross-sectional triangular shape as the missing natural tooth did not benefit the aesthetic outcome to a great extent (as it is supposed to do) due to the nature of the peri-implant soft tissue. When an anatomical abutment is used, it will give the required original missing tooth configuration at the emergence level while it is in place, but upon its removal for any clinical reason, the peri-implant soft tissue tends to collapse and regain its original circular shape. Therefore, the final prosthesis that possesses natural biological contours seems to fulfill the same purpose without the need for the use of anatomical abutments. With regard to which implant type permits ease of control of apicoincisal positioning,

the screw design ranks first: its mechanical character allows control of the depth while threading the fixture in the bone. The cylinder design, on the other hand, requires the use of an implant retrieval tool to adjust the implant's optimal vertical position, which makes the procedure difficult to control. Additionally, implants with wide diameters of 5–6 mm will eventually require less space for transitioning into a natural tooth form than narrow-diameter implants (Fig. 3.19).

It is recommended that the location of the implant neck should be related to a line connecting the gingival zenith of the adjacent remaining natural dentition rather than to a line connecting the CEJ or the crest of the ridge. Therefore, when the implant-supported restoration is completed, it will attain the same marginal level as those existing around natural dentition. The gingival zenith is not a constant reference point; it sometimes moves apically in case of recession, and it reflects the actual clinical marginal level of the

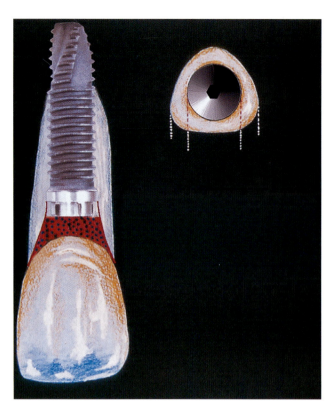

FIGURE 3.17. Illustration showing the difference in cross section between implant and natural tooth and the running room.

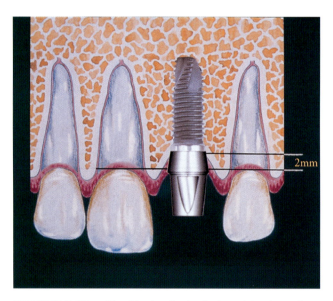

FIGURE 3.18. The ideal apicoincisal positioning of the implant.

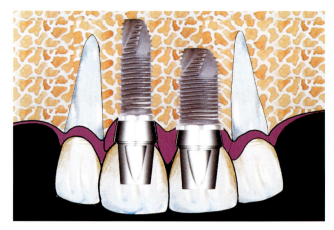

FIGURE 3.19. Illustration showing that wider implants require less apical positioning.

a wavy course that has a rise and fall on both buccolingual and interproximal margins; this scalloped line does not move when gingival recession occurs.

The crest of the ridge also is not an ideal reference point, since the very nature of bone resorption makes it sometimes variable in its height, and also the soft tissue thickness on top of it can be variable. For that reason, when implant placement is in an area afflicted with mild vertical ridge resorption and a remarkably thick mucosa, the implant neck should be situated above the level of the bone crest in order to keep the "running room" within the required average level (2–3 mm). On the other hand, in restoration of a missing single tooth for a patient that exhibits nonpathological gingival recession, the only ideal reference line will be the line connecting the gingival zeniths of the adjacent teeth.

Lastly, there is a relationship between the apicoincisal and labiopalatal positioning. Labiopalatal placement of the implant is directly proportional to its apicoincisal positioning. Potashnick stated that, for every millimeter the implant is placed palatally, the implant should be sunken 1 mm apically for compensation, in order to maintain a natural emergence profile.[5] This relationship was found to be helpful in obtaining an optimal implant position.[5]

CORRECTIONS OF IMPLANT MISPLACEMENT

Any deviation from the optimal position of the implant in any dimension will surely result in an aesthetic problem. Some of the problems can be treated, while for others, implant removal will be the only possible resort. An implant that is placed in an incorrect position in the alveolar ridge may be due to the use of an imprecise surgical template, instability of the angulation of the handpiece, and the lack of knowledge or experience. As in the case of

soft tissue at the time of implant placement. In contrast, the CEJ is a constant landmark. It follows a uniformly fixed scalloped path along the root surface. It also pursues any positioning error, there is always a consequence or repercussion. Therefore, it is essential that the clinician should be familiar with the various unfortunate clinical situations that may arise in order to be able to deal with them.

The problem associated with positioning the implant too far apically is the formation of a deep gingival sulcus. This creates a favorable environment for several types of bacteria, including anaerobic bacteria, to colonize and populate, due to the inaccessibility for cleaning (Fig. 3.20).[17] Gingival bleeding upon tooth brushing or when the prosthetic components are to be retrieved is a common event with too far apical placement. Moreover, accessibility to the prosthetic margins of a deeply seated implant becomes difficult, especially when the restoration is to be cemented. It becomes increasingly exigent to ensure complete removal of the luting cement from the interface between the abutment and the restoration.[40] The correction of this clinical dilemma is almost impossible because gingival recession usually occurs as a result; strict oral hygiene procedures should be maintained to reduce the tendency for gingival inflammation.

The implant placed too far incisally, in contrast, often results in a short crown with constricted margins due to the reduced space for "running room." This makes stacking the prosthetic components difficult. This clinical predicament is impossible to amend or rectify. The difficulty remains in handling the margins of the final prosthesis and hiding the abutment collar sublingually (Fig. 3.21). In this particular condition, implant removal can be the treatment of choice.

The chances to restore a misplaced implant with an acceptable aesthetic result are minimal. This is especially the case if the implant has been positioned too far labially

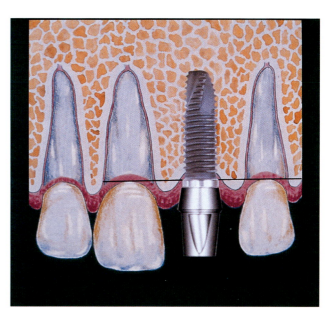

FIGURE 3.21. Too far incisal positioning of an implant fixture.

or incisally. Even using the pre-angulated abutments in too far labial implant placement will not be effective in most situations because the pre-angled abutment usually requires a larger restorative dimension than other types. The protruding gingival collar of the pre-angled abutment will encroach upon the peri-implant soft tissue and violate its integrity. Interestingly, Nishimura et al. have described an alternative approach for patients with misplaced dental implants that are difficult to restore with the regular commercially available abutments.[41] This approach suggests the use of a custom-fabricated abutment that is specially designed to meet the aesthetic and functional needs of each particular patient.

Other attempts have been made to correct implant misplacement by performing an osteotomy around the osseous housing of the implant fixture, moving the segment to the required correct position, and stabilizing it with microplates and screws.[42] This procedure can save the patient the distress of going through several surgical procedures to remove the misplaced implant and replace it, which involves longer treatment time. This technique has its limitations: limited space between the existing natural root and the implant fixture that sometimes makes the osteotomy clinically inapplicable; insufficient keratinized tissues to cover the surgical site; anatomical limitations; and risk of morbidity or other unforeseen surgical difficulties. However, despite all these hindrances, sometimes removal of the implant may be the only reliable solution to treat implant misplacement.

In conclusion, the balance between function and aesthetics must be maintained, and since delicate viable tissue is being dealt with in the oral cavity, the necessity to achieve accurate and precise implant placement is empha-

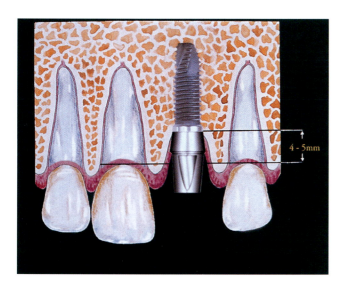

FIGURE 3.20. Too far apical placement of an implant fixture; note the increased pocket depth.

sized. Tipping of the balance is a price that cannot be paid!

REFERENCES

1. English CE. Biomechanical concerns with fixed partial dentures involving implants. Implant Dent 1993(2): 221–242.
2. Atwood DA and Coy DA. Clinical, cephalometric and densitometric study of reduction of residual ridge. J Prosthet Dent 1971(26): 280–293.
3. Johnson K. A study of the dimensional changes occurring in the maxilla after tooth extraction. Part I: Normal healing. Aust Dent J 1963(8): 428–433.
4. Carlsson GE, Bergman B, and Headegard B. Changes in contour of the maxillary alveolar process under immediate dentures. A longitudinal clinical and x-ray cephalometric study covering 5 years. Acta Odontol Scand 1967(25): 45–75.
5. Potashnick SR. Soft tissue modeling for the esthetic single-tooth implant restoration. J Esthet Dent 1998(10): 121–131.
6. Jansen CE and Weisgold A. Presurgical treatment planning for the anterior single-tooth implant restoration. Compendium 1995(16): 746–763.
7. Chiche GJ and Aoshima H. Functional versus aesthetic articulation of maxillary anterior restorations. Pract Periodont Aesthet Dent 1997(9): 335–342.
8. Spiekerman HS. Special diagnostic methods for implant patients. In Implantology. Stuttgart: Thieme Verlag, 1995, 91–124.
9. Garber DA. The esthetic dental implant: Letting the restoration be the guide. J Am Dent Assoc 1995(126): 319–325.
10. Palacci P. Optimal implant positioning. In Palacci P and Ericsson I. Esthetic Implant Dentistry. Soft and Hard Tissue Management. Berlin: Quintessence Publishing Co., 2001, 101–135.
11. Buser D, Mericske-Stern R, Dula K, and Lang NP. Clinical experience with one-stage, non-submerged dental implants. Adv Dent Res 1999(13): 153–161.
12. Burger EH and Klein-Nulend J. Responses of bone cells to biomechanical forces in vitro. Adv Dent Res 1999(13): 93–98.
13. Herrmann G. Primary stability of oral implants. Int Mag Oral Implantol 2000(1): 22–24.
14. Szmukler-Moncler S, Salama H, Reingewirtz Y, and Dubruille JH. Timing of loading and effect of micromotion on bone-dental implant interface: Review of experimental literature. J Biomed Mater Res 1998(43): 192–203.
15. Block MS, Kent JN, and Guerra LR. Implants in Dentistry. Philadelphia: W. B. Saunders Co., 1997.
16. Brunski JB, Puleo DA, and Nanci A. Biomaterials and biomechanics of oral and maxillofacial implants: Current status and future developments. Int J Oral Maxillofac Implants 2000(15): 15–46.
17. Misch CE. The maxillary anterior single tooth implant aesthetic health compromise, . Int J Dent Symp 1995 (1):4–9 .
18. El Askary AS, Meffert RM, and Griffin T. Why do dental implants fail? Part I. Implant Dent 1999(8): 173–185.
19. El Askary AS, Meffert RM, and Griffin T. Why do Dental Implants Fail? Part II. Implant Dent 1999(8): 265–277.
20. Meffert RM. Treatment of failing dental implants. Curr Opin Dent 1992(2): 109–144.
21. Seibrt J. Surgical management of osseous defects. In Gorman HM and Cohen DW, eds. Periodontal Therapy, 5th ed. St. Louis: CV Mosby Co., 1973, 765–766.
22. Oschsenbein C and Ross S. A concept of osseous surgery and its clinical applications. In Ward HL and Chas C eds. A Periodontal Point of View. Springfield, IL: Charles C. Thomas, 1973).
23. Olsson M and Lindhe J. Periodontal characteristics in individuals with varying forms of the upper central incisors. J Clin Periodontol 1991(18): 78–82.
24. Morris ML. The position of the margin of the gingiva. Oral Surg Oral Med Oral Pathol 1958(11): 722–734.
25. Wheeler RC. Complete crown form and the periodontium. J Prosthet Dent 1961(11): 722–734.
26. Wheeler RC. A Text Book of Dental Anatomy and Physiology, 2nd ed. Philadelphia: W. B. Saunders Co, 1950.
27. Glickman I. Clinical Periodontology, 4th ed. Philadelphia: W. B. Saunders Co., 1972, 21.
28. Seibert J and Lindhe J. Esthetics and periodontal therapy. In Lindhe J, ed. Text Book of Clinical Periodontology, 2nd ed. Copenhagen: Munksgaard, 1988.
29. Zitzman NU and Marinello CP. Anterior single-tooth replacement: Clinical examination and treatment planning. Pract Periodont Aesthet Dent 1999(11): 847–858.
30. Esposito M, Ekestubbe A, and Grondah K. Radiological evaluation of marginal bone loss at tooth surfaces facing single Branemark implants. Clin Oral Impl Res 1993(4): 151–157.
31. Jansen CE. Restorative options with implant dentistry. J Calif Dent Assoc 1992(20): 30–31.
32. El Askary AS. Esthetic considerations in anterior single-tooth replacement. Implant Dent 1999(8): 61–67.
33. Kennedy B.D, Collins TA, and Kline PC. Simplified guide for precise implant placement: A technical note. Int J Oral Maxillofac Implants 1998(13): 684–688.
34. Ohenell L, Palmquist J, and Brånemark PI. Single tooth replacement. In Worthington P and Brånemark P-I, eds. Advanced Osseointegration Surgery Applications in the Maxillofacial Region. Carol Stream, IL: Quintessence Publishing Co., 1992, 211–232.
35. Askary AS. Why do dental implants fail? Part I. Implant Dent 1999(8): 173–185.
36. Parel SM and Sulivan DY. Esthetics and Osseointegration. Dallas, TX: Taylor Publishing, 1989.
37. Daftary F. Natural esthetics with implant prosthesis. J Esthet Dent 1995(7): 9–17.
38. Davidoff D. Developing soft tissue contours for implant supported restorations: A simplified method for enhanced aesthetics. Pract Periodont Aesthet Dent 1996(8): 507–513.
39. Wheeler RC. Dental Anatomy, Physiology and Occlusion. 5th ed. Philadelphia: W. B. Saunders Co., 1974.

40. Agar J, Cameron S, Hughbanks J, and Parker M. Cement removal from restorations luted to titanium abutments with simulated subgingival margins. J Prosthet Dent 1997(78): 43–47.

41. Nishimura RD, Chang TL, Perri GR, et al. Restoration of partially edentulous patients using customized implant abutements. Pract Periodont Aesthet Dent 1999(11): 669–676.

42. Warden P J . Surgical repositioning of a malposed, unserviceable implant: Case report. Int J Oral Maxillofac Surg 2000(58): 433–435.

4
Soft Tissue Management

Abd El Salam El Askary

The soft tissue in the oral cavity may be likened to an outer frame that magnifies and complements the beauty of the natural teeth within. Without this outer frame the color, contrast, and luster of the teeth will not attain maximum attractiveness. If one were to imagine the teeth without the surrounding soft tissue, one would be aghast at the image of just teeth coming out of the bone. That image is one that shows how important the soft tissue is, in simply giving life to the total image. It is this total image of teeth with healthy surrounding soft tissue that clinicians seek to replicate in oral implantology to give a natural tooth appearance.

The soft tissue that closely surrounds the implant collar (the peri-implant soft tissue) is delicate in nature. Understandably, it is impossible to achieve satisfactory aesthetic results without peri-implant soft tissue that is harmonious with the adjacent tissues in color, form, and contour.[1,2] Peri-implant architecture thus takes a major share in the aesthetic setup of any implant-supported restoration.[3–6]

Currently available soft tissue manipulations of the peri-implant soft tissue can solve a number of minor clinical problems that prosthetic simulated soft tissue restorations attempted to handle in the past. For example, connective tissue grafts can amend minor alveolar ridge defects and restore original contours by increasing the soft tissue height and width.[7–9] Soft tissue expansion by means of a provisional restoration is yet another modern application in soft tissue management; it is used to enhance the aesthetic outcome or help solve an existing soft tissue clinical problem.[10,11] A provisional restoration also can compensate for a palatally positioned implant by expanding the peri-implant soft tissue margin in a labial direction until it levels and harmonizes with the adjacent tissues.[12–14]

Unlike the natural dentition, a dental implant is a metallic body inserted into the jawbone. Therefore, its collar does not receive any blood supply from a surrounding periodontal ligament or any other vessels. Rather, it acquires a fibrous connective tissue band around its collar that is more dense and acellular.[15–19] In addition, the very fragile nature of the oral mucosa makes its ability to withstand excessive clinical manipulations unpredictable, which can lead sometimes to asymmetrical final implant prostheses (Fig. 4.1).[20] In view of the above, clinicians are required to handle peri-implant soft tissues with exceptional care because of their reduced blood circulation and delicate nature. Mastering the techniques of manipulating the delicate peri-implant soft tissue architecture in the aesthetic zone is therefore considered mandatory. It can lead to a remarkable improvement in the aesthetic outcome of implant-supported restorations when the other treatment steps are properly fulfilled.

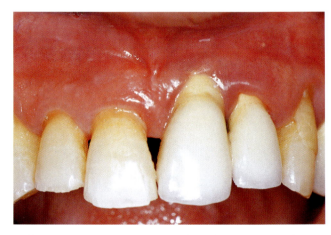

FIGURE 4.1. Nonsymmetrical implant-supported restoration, due to soft tissue mismanagement.

Aesthetic implant positioning has a direct influence on the soft tissue profile and final appearance.[21] The more precisely the implant is positioned, the easier it will be to obtain a natural-looking, implant-supported restoration in its soft tissue housing. With optimal implant positioning, any gingival discrepancy will be avoided, thus minimizing the need for further corrective surgeries and soft tissue reconstruction.

Accurate diagnosis and treatment planning set the stage for the timing of all the events to follow. This has its direct impact on the precision of the work and the predictability of the final results. It is important to be able to identify and classify the existing clinical conditions, whether they are related to hard or soft tissue origin.

Ridge defects have a wide range of descriptions with numerous variations in size, severity, and extent. Allen et al. identified three categories of ridge defects in relation to the healthy soft tissue margins: (a) mild, a defect of less than 3 mm; (b) moderate, a defect of 3–6 mm; and (c) severe, a defect greater than 6 mm.[22] Seibert and Salama, on the other hand, classified volumetric deformity changes of the edentulous ridge into three general categories: Class I, buccolingual loss of tissue with normal ridge height in an apicocoronal dimension; Class II, apicocoronal loss of tissue with normal ridge width in a buccolingual dimension; and Class III, combination buccolingual and apicocoronal loss of tissue, resulting in loss of normal ridge height and width.[23] These classifications not only facilitate the assessment of any given clinically compromised situation, but also help the dental team to identify the existing soft tissue status and describe it in a more specific and scientific manner that contributes to better communication among the dental team.

In many situations, after classifying the existing hard and/or soft tissue defects, the clinician may have to resort to surgical reconstruction of these tissues from the outset. The surgical reconstruction enables the clinician to restore the alveolar ridge to its original biological dimensions. This, in turn, will help the clinician to restore the missing dentition with greater precision and predictability. It is important to note, however, that these cosmetic surgical procedures may result in additional discomfort and financial cost for the patient as well as additional chair time for the dentist.

TIMING IN RELATION TO SOFT TISSUE MANAGEMENT

There is no specific time when management of peri-implant soft tissue should take place. Proactive soft tissue management can be performed throughout the various stages of implant treatment. Soft tissue can be influenced during many stages of implant treatment. The second-stage surgery is an example where the labial mucosa exists in a collapsed state.[20] It would require support from the prosthetic components to develop natural-looking peri-implant soft tissue contours. Mucogingival surgical corrections can also be used before or after implant placement to reconstruct the missing aesthetic biological contours surrounding already existing implant-supported restorations.[24–26]

Correction of edentulous ridge defects can be performed at any time during the period of the treatment plan. Soft tissue correction of a deficient edentulous ridge is best performed before implant placement; this can help improve aesthetics, phonetics, and oral hygiene maintenance.[27] Soft tissue management at the time of tooth extraction can be determinative to the final aesthetic outcome as well. Soft tissue refining and profiling, on the other hand, are intermediate clinical procedures in implant treatment that can be executed after the abutment connection.

The time allowed for soft tissue healing after cosmetic reconstruction is important. Lazara recommends that consideration should be given to the healing period after any soft tissue manipulation occurred, as oral soft tissues require an ample time to heal and mend.[28] A stable soft tissue clinical condition must be attained before beginning or continuing with other clinical procedures. This is also reaffirmed by Small and Tarnow, who recommend a three-month waiting period for the soft tissue to stabilize before selecting the final abutment or making the final impression after the second-stage surgery.[29]

In their longitudinal study of gingival recession around dental implants, Small and Tarnow measured the soft tissue level around implants following surgery to determine if a predictable pattern of soft tissue changes could be identified. They evaluated sixty-three implants in eleven patients. Baseline measurements were recorded at the second-stage surgery in two different submerged implant systems. Subsequent measurements were recorded at one week, one month, three months, six months, nine months, and one year after baseline measurements. The majority of the recession occurred within the first three months, and 80% of all sites exhibited recession on the buccal surface. It is therefore recommended to allow three months time for the tissue to stabilize and mature before either selecting a final abutment or making a final impression in order to avoid any unpredictable tissue behavior around the final prosthesis.[29]

The author has classified management of the soft tissues around dental implants in the aesthetic zone according to the timing of clinical intervention into four categories: (1) before implant placement, (2) during implant placement, (3) at the time of abutment connection, and (4) at postabutment connection.[30]

Soft Tissue Management before Implant Placement

After the future surgical site for implant placement is carefully examined in order to identify any defects or discrepancies in the keratinized band. Any corrective soft tissue surgery (if needed) should be performed two to four months before the first-stage implant placement surgery takes place, to allow ample time for the soft tissue to reach a stable remodeling state, as mentioned earlier.[31]

Soft tissue therapy prior to implant placement utilizes various techniques to enhance the quantity or the quality of the soft tissue or to eliminate any existing soft tissue pathology at the area of interest. Free gingival grafting,[32] connective tissue grafting,[33] or a combination of both can also be used at this stage to enhance the final aesthetic results as well as minimize the complications that might arise at the time of the first- and second-stage surgeries.[34]

The methods of dealing with the soft tissue before implant placement follow below.

OPTIMIZING KERATINIZED TISSUES The general biological nature of the oral mucosa is fragility. The mucosa can be easily torn and traumatized during intraoperative procedures, leading to postoperative sloughing and a subsequent delay in healing that might jeopardize the future aesthetics. This explains the need to improve the soft tissue status prior to surgery.

Improving the condition of the keratinized mucosa prior to implant surgery can be a safeguard for the future health of the implant and its surrounding tissues. Presence of a sufficient zone of keratinized mucosa can minimize the soft tissue manipulations (especially in immediate implant placements) needed to achieve primary closure over the future implant site.

Immediate implant placement into a freshly extracted socket presents an especially difficult challenge to achieving soft tissue coverage, especially with patients that have the thin scalloped tissue biotype. To overcome these clinical difficulties, a technique for developing keratinized tissues on top of the socket orifice has been introduced.[35] The technique entails the use of a round bur to reduce the tooth height below the crestal bone level without traumatizing the surrounding gingival margin.[35] The presence of residual roots of the reduced teeth will prevent epithelial downgrowth along the socket walls and provide scaffolding for the regeneration of keratinized tissues on top of the socket orifice. The soft tissues will take only few weeks to regenerate and fill the socket orifice as part of the healing process.

This technique provides sufficient keratinized mucosa for a soft tissue closure procedure on top of the implant. This new regenerated tissue subsequently minimizes surgical trauma that occurs due to attempts to achieve primary closure in immediate implant placement. In addition, the new regenerated tissue preserves the anatomical mucogingival integrity at its biological level (Fig. 4.2a–e) and eliminates the chance for postextraction alveolar bone resorption.[36–38]

Generally speaking, the regenerated oral tissues should be in excess of what is required so as to compensate for ensuing tissue shrinkage or remodeling[39,40] (especially following multiple surgical interventions). After sufficient healing time has elapsed and a stable tissue contour is established, any excessive tissue can then be trimmed or sculptured to the desired level.

SOCKET SEAL TECHNIQUES This technique is used prior to implant placement to improve the condition of the soft tissue on top of the socket orifice, to prevent postextraction bone resorption of the alveolar

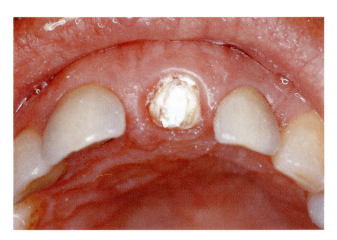

FIGURE 4.2a. A patient with unsalvageable remaining root of the maxillary left central incisor.

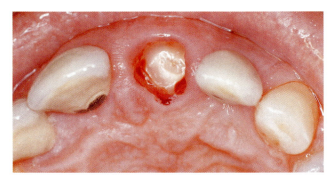

FIGURE 4.2b. Reduction of the root level below the crest of the alveolar bone with a rose-head bur.

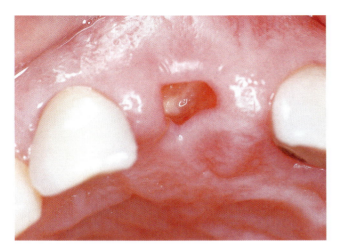

FIGURE 4.2c. A four weeks postoperative view showing regeneration of new keratinized tissues.

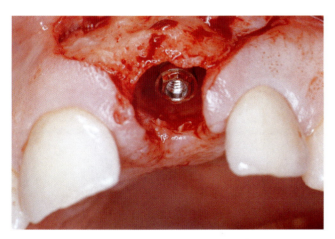

FIGURE 4.2d. Clinical view after root extraction, showing reflection of the muccoperiosteal flap with the implant in place.

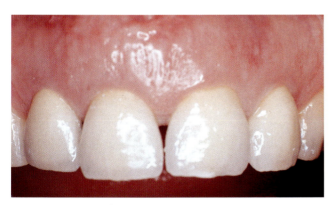

FIGURE 4.2e. Postinsertion view of the final restoration in place, showing an excellent soft tissue condition with zero scar tissues.

ridge, and to enhance the quality of bone at the future implant site. The technique of socket sealing aims to block off the socket of an extracted tooth immediately after tooth extraction. Socket seal surgery was first described by Landsberg[41] and Bichacho[42] as a treatment method for preserving the integrity of the alveolar ridge and inhibiting apical epithelial migration into the socket.[43]

The procedure involves atraumatic, flapless tooth extraction, followed by debridement and decortication of the socket walls to enhance osteogenic activity. The free gingival margins surrounding the socket are circumferentially deepithelialized with a water-cooled, round coarse diamond bur or with a sharp scalpel in order to provide vascularity for the future free gingival graft and to promote clot formation. The socket is then packed with the bone graft of choice.

Since any bone-grafting material must be kept in place and protected from the hostile oral environment,[43] a 3 mm thick free gingival graft is harvested from the palate to cover the bone-grafting material. The free gingival graft is then adapted and fitted to the freshly deepithelialized gingival margins on top of the bone graft and sutured, to completely seal the socket orifice. The purpose of the socket sealing technique is to prevent physical, chemical, or bacterial contamination of the organizing blood clot and bone-grafting material until healing occurs (Fig 4.3a–c).

The technique is considered to be a simple clinical procedure that can be performed along with tooth extraction. However, this technique has its shortcomings. The soft tissue graft lies on the bone graft particles and not on the periosteum. Therefore, the surrounding gingival tissue located on the rim of the socket becomes the only source of vascularity to the free gingival graft. As a result, the soft tissue graft is prone to thinning, necrosis, and infection, due to the poor blood supply to the graft. If the

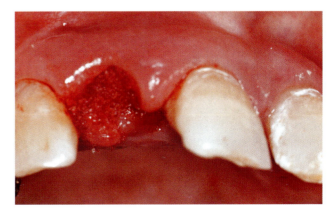

FIGURE 4.3a. The socket condition after tooth extraction and bone grafting.

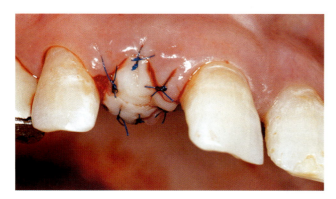

FIGURE 4.3b. Keratinized tissue graft is adapted and sutured to the socket orifice.

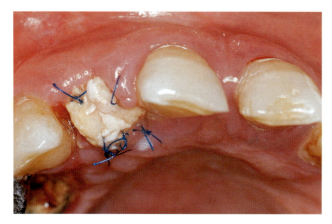

FIGURE 4.3c. Unfavorable graft healing occurred (sloughing) due to decreased blood supply to the graft.

soft tissue graft survives, it generally does not come to possess the same texture or color as the surrounding soft tissues.

MODIFIED SOCKET SEAL SURGERY Misch et al. have modified the previously mentioned technique of socket sealing in order to eliminate its drawbacks and improve its clinical predictability.[44] The modified socket seal surgery is performed prior to implant placement in order to enhance the quantity and quality of bone and soft tissue as well as to preserve the original biological architecture of the alveolar ridge at the place of tooth extraction. It is preferably performed when the socket walls are intact. In this technique, a composite graft, consisting of epithelial tissue, connective tissue, periosteum, cortical bone, and cancellous bone, is harvested from the tuberosity area to fill and seal the socket. There are several advantages to using a composite graft. For one, the connective tissue part of the graft has an advantage over the keratinized tissue graft: it merges and blends with the adjacent keratinized tissues after completion of the healing process, providing keratinized

epithelium on top of the socket with an exact color and texture similar to that of the surrounding original tissues. Also, the use of the autogenous bone is found to be more predictable for bone regenerative procedures.[45–47] Misch et al.[44] have also used platelet-derived growth factor (PDGF) from the patient's own blood that functions as a chemoattractant for mesenchymal cells to enhance cartilage and bone formation rate.[48]

The procedure entails a flapless atraumatic extraction of the unsalvageable tooth, followed by curettage and decortication of the socket walls, and the soft tissue around the rim of the extraction socket is then deepithelialized with a diamond bur or a sharp scalpel (Fig. 4.4a–c). A trephine drill that has a diameter almost the same as or larger than that of the socket orifice is used to harvest the composite graft from the tuberosity. Care must be exercised not to cause excessive heat generation to the

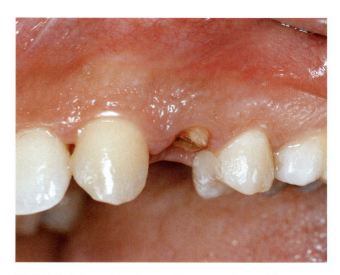

FIGURE 4.4a. A patient with an unsalvageable remaining root of the maxillary first premolar.

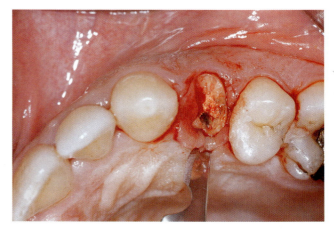

FIGURE 4.4b. Deepithelialization of the soft tissue margins.

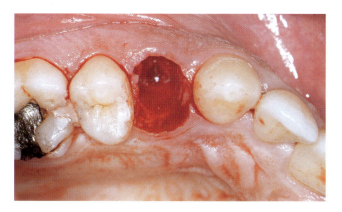

FIGURE 4.4c. Flapless atraumatic extraction of the remaining root with intact labial plate of bone.

graft. This is accomplished by using a slow-speed handpiece with copious saline irrigation during the harvesting procedure.

A green stick fracture of the composite graft is performed at its base to separate it from the donor site. Here, caution must be exercised not to perforate the maxillary sinus; an x-ray film or digital radiography can help determine the extent of drilling procedure (Fig. 4.4d,e). The keratinized layer of the graft core is then shaved to remove only the surface epithelium, leaving almost 3 mm of connective tissue thickness attached to the bone core (Fig. 4.4f). If the bone core is found to be larger than the socket orifice, it should be pared so that it will fit snugly in the socket. The apical third of the extraction socket is subsequently filled with demineralized freeze-dried bone and

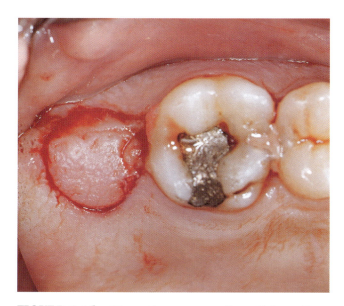

FIGURE 4.4d. Harvesting a composite graft from the maxillary tuberosity region using a wide trephine drill that is almost the same diameter as the socket orifice.

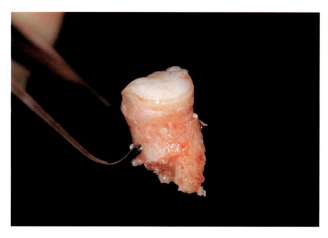

FIGURE 4.4e. The composite graft after harvesting (cancellous bone, connective tissue, and keratinized tissue).

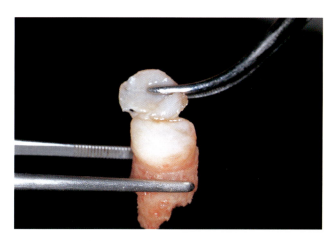

FIGURE 4.4f. Removal of the keratinized epithelium from the composite graft.

a puffy coat containing PDGF (Fig. 4.4g). Afterwards the composite graft is introduced into the socket (Fig. 4.4h) and tapped gently into place using a mallet and blunt instrument. Upon seating, the surface of the composite graft should conform to the crestal contour of the socket and be positioned slightly below the surrounding marginal gingiva (Fig. 4.4i). This is to allow for epithelial migration on top of the connective tissue graft. The connective tissue portion of the graft is then sutured to the surrounding gingival tissues (Fig. 4.4j).

When this technique is used, a provisional removable prosthesis should not be allowed during the first few weeks after surgery because the composite graft may move upon pressure and become sequestered due to premature loading of the bone resulting from the pressure of fitting surface of the prosthesis. The osteotomy hole of the donor site can be filled with any bone-grafting material,

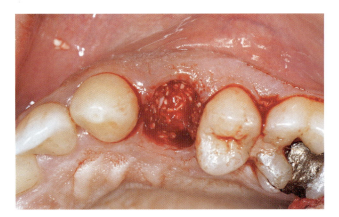

FIGURE 4.4g. Condensation of freeze-dried bone inside the apical third of the socket.

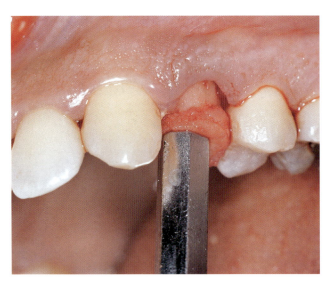

FIGURE 4.4h. The prepared graft is being introduced into the socket and tapped.

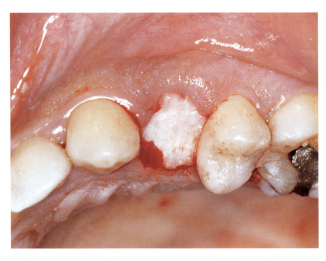

FIGURE 4.4i. The graft is positioned below the gingival margin to allow epithelial growth on its surface.

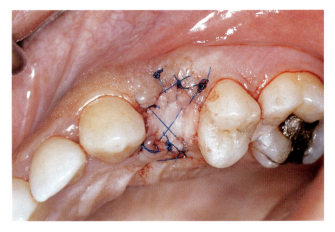

FIGURE 4.4j. The graft is sutured in its final placement.

and primary wound closure can be achieved by undermining the soft tissue edges, or an acrylic template may be used to seal the area of the defect until it heals by secondary intention.

The numerous advantages of this technique include the great enhancement of the soft tissue quality and quantity over the socket (which attains the exact color and texture of the surrounding tissues) (Fig. 4.4k) and the promotion of faster and more predictable bone regeneration in the socket (Fig. 4.4l), so that the width and height of the alveolar bone are maintained after extraction (Fig. 4.4m), thus improving the overall prognosis for any future implant placement. This method is considered a highly predictable technique among all the techniques used to enhance socket condition prior to implant therapy (Fig. 4.4n).

Soft Tissue Management during Implant Placement

Surgical techniques utilized during implant placement at the first-stage surgery are numerous; the techniques

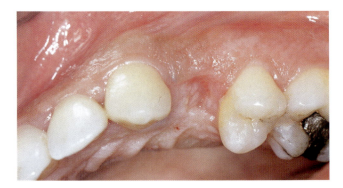

FIGURE 4.4k. Healing of the area with the contour of the labial plate of bone intact and with no postoperative resorption (note the color match of the soft tissue part of the graft to the surrounding tissues).

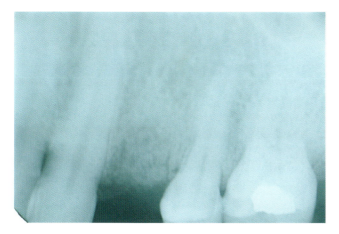

FIGURE 4.4l.   Periapical radiographic view of the area showing bone regeneration in the socket with improved bone density.

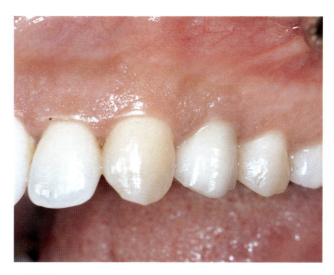

FIGURE 4.4n.   Post crown insertion view.

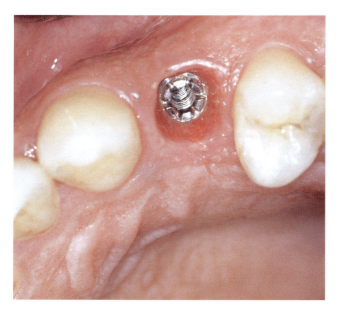

FIGURE 4.4m.   The final soft tissue healing after the second-stage surgery with the contour of the labial plate of bone intact.

should all aim at fulfilling the standard operative recommendations in mucoperiosteal flap management as well as closure. Incision design, mucoperiosteal flap handling, careful soft tissue manipulation, and tension-free flap closure contribute to providing a healthy environment around dental implants and minimizing postoperative complications.[49–51] The first-stage surgery involves the placement of the dental implant either in an immediate or a delayed fashion.[52,53] Surgical procedures utilized to achieve delayed implant placement will surely differ from those used in immediate placement, and postoperative soft tissue healing will accordingly not be the same.

On the other hand, nonsubmerged implant placement requires a different surgical approach than submerged implant placement. Nonsubmerged implant placement does not require a second-stage surgery because the access to the implant is maintained above the soft tissue from the time of its placement.[54–56] Buser et al.[54] stated that osseointegration showed high predictability in the one-stage, nonsubmerged surgical protocol; this referred to the elimination of the subgingival implant-abutment connections. However, it is the author's opinion that when aesthetics is a priority, the nonsubmerged one-stage implant placement protocol should be restricted. The reasoning is grounded in the inherent character of the design of the one-stage implant system. The flaring of the transmucosal part of the implant handicaps the use of the provisional restoration to develop the "running room" within which the natural emergence through the soft tissues can be replicated. The nonsubmerged (two-stage) implant placement protocol entails the attachment of the healing abutment to the implant fixture at the time of implant insertion; the implant is permitted to heal in a nonsubmerged mode to provide greater latitude for proper soft tissue contouring. However, submerging the implant beneath the soft tissue for a two-stage surgical protocol is still the method most preferred by clinicians, probably because there is extensive long-term documentation in the literature[57] and the implant is not subjected to any biting loads while it is undergoing osseointegration.[58–60]

The standard submerged protocol for placing dental implants might be indicated when the aesthetic outcome of the implant restoration is significantly important, when the implant is placed in poor bone quality or in a site that has been previously augmented, and when periodontal therapy has not been concluded at the time of implant placement.

SOFT TISSUE MANAGEMENT IN DELAYED IMPLANT PLACEMENT

Mucoperiosteal Flap Design Flap design is an important clinical step in dental implant placement; some clinicians prefer to design the flap in the presurgical stage on the study cast because of its value in the success of the treatment. The flap should be designed to gain access and visibility with minimal soft tissue trauma and to facilitate maintenance of the attached tissues. This in turn will help achieve favorable healing and minimize postoperative complications.[61–64]

The concept behind selecting one flap design over another is mainly to achieve optimal wound healing that contributes positively to implant survival.[65] Because the oral cavity harbors numerous microorganisms, it becomes a hostile environment for dental implants, especially in the healing period.[66] Therefore, placing a dental implant in such an environment warrants special attention. Esposito et al. expressed an important fact that links wound healing with implant survival; he stated that clinical signs of oral tissue infection during the postoperative period of a submerged implant insertion can indicate an increased risk of implant failure.[67] Systemic conditions such as uncontrolled diabetes mellitus, severe anemia, uremia, and jaundice can also be considered aggravating factors that impair wound healing.[65] Therefore, special emphasis should be directed towards delicate soft tissue manipulation and handling.

Obviously, there is no strict recommendation in the literature for selecting a particular flap design over another; the incision and flap design are usually selected according to the clinician's preference following the rule that says, "Whatever works best in the clinician's hands works best for the patient." However, the general health condition of the patient, quality and quantity of the keratinized soft tissues, tissue biotype, width of the vestibule, presence of osseous defects, the design of the implant used, and the location of anatomical landmarks are all factors that must be considered when choosing any flap design.

There are several flap designs used for dental implant placement with various surgical approaches. The classic vestibular approach to accessing the alveolar ridge in implant placement surgery was first described by Brånemark et al.[53,57] The design involves a horizontal incision in the vestibular mucosa parallel to the gingival margin. A lingually or palatally pedicled mucoperiosteal flap is next obtained through two vertical incisions. The objective of this design is to position the incision line away from the head of the implants. This particular approach has several disadvantages, especially in patients with shallow vestibules. These disadvantages include severe postoperative edema and compromised blood supply to

the site accompanied by an inflammatory reaction (which can be a potential risk of infection).[68]

Another flap design for submerged implant placement is the crestal approach. This approach has shown many advantages. It is simple, does not require professional surgical experience, can be easily sutured, offers faster healing, does not compromise the blood supply to the site, and exhibits a mild inflammatory reaction.[68,69]

Various studies have been conducted to judge the efficacy of vestibular versus crestal approaches used for submerged dental implant placement. A study by Casino et al. compared the vestibular and crestal approaches in relation to the success rate of osseointegration. The clinical success of osseointegration was evaluated at the second-stage surgery.[70] In this study, a crestal incision was used for 1,705 implants in 381 patients, and a vestibular approach was used for placing 593 implants in 141 patients. The outcome showed no statistically significant difference in the clinical success of osseointegration between the two approaches.

A similar retrospective study by Scharf and Tarnow weighed the clinical success rate of osseointegrated implants at the time of the second-stage surgery using the same two surgical approaches.[68] A total of 386 implants was placed in 92 patients; 265 implants were placed in 60 patients using a vestibular incision and showed a success rate of 98.8%; 121 implants were placed in 32 patients using a crestal incision and showed a success rate of 98.3%. They concluded that there was no statistically significant difference in the success rates of dental implants between the vestibular incision and crestal incision approaches.

Another study by Hunt attempted to demonstrate which incision, crestal or vestibular, is more suitable for placing dental implants.[71] Hunt also found that no single flap design was optimal for implant surgery.[71] More importantly, he recommended that basic factors like flap design, blood supply, visibility, access, atraumatic handling, and primary tension-free closure on healthy bone be carefully considered in implant placement.

Preservative Interproximal Papilla Incision

Aesthetic and functional placement of dental implants requires a flap design that provides accessibility, visibility, and workability without jeopardizing soft tissue health or integrity. Including the interproximal papillae in the mucoperiosteal flap is not recommended in aesthetic areas; therefore, excluding the interproximal papillae from the mucoperiosteal flap will help to achieve good aesthetic results. Some authors stated that raising the interproximal papillae along with the rest of the mucoperiosteal flap might lead to an unpleasant aesthetic outcome.[72,73] This can be related to the tendency of the soft tissue to shrink or recede after raising a mucoperiosteal flap, because a slight bone resorption occurs each time a full mucoperiosteal flap is raised.[74]

It is the author's experience that the preservative interproximal papilla approach during the first- and/or second-stage surgery will favor aesthetics because the preservation of the papillae stabilizes the adjacent margins of the implant-supported prosthesis, reduces postoperative soft tissue recession, and reduces the tendency for marginal bone loss (Fig. 4.5a,b).[75,76]

An added advantage to the flap design that safeguards the interproximal papillae is a lessened tendency to lacerate the interdental papillae during surgery. The smaller size of the interproximal papillae, added to their delicate nature, makes them easy to tear or lacerate during the different stages in flap handling.

The preservative interproximal papilla flap design allows better flap adaptation upon closure; in other words, when the preservative design is used, each vertical incision of the mucoperiosteal flap meets with the adjacent tissues in a soft-tissue-to-soft-tissue manner (at the mesiocervical angle of the adjacent natural teeth), while in nonpreservative flap designs, the vertical incision rests on the mesiocervical aspect of the tooth structure; therefore, the preservative design adapts in a soft-tissue-to-soft-tissue manner, while the nonpreservative design adapts in a soft-tissue-to-tooth manner at the mesiocervical area.

The preservative interproximal papilla flap design can be used in several clinical applications; it can be used in placing dental implants routinely, at the second-stage surgery, and in bone-grafting procedures.

Modified Elden-Mejchar Technique
The modified Elden-Mejchar technique is a flap design that is used for implant placement to create an optimal mucosal condition with maximum stability and reduced pocket depth around dental implants. The flap design

can be used as an alternative to the classic full thickness mucoperiosteal design used for submerged implant placement. The original Elden-Mejchar[77] vestibuloplasty was modified by Hertel[78] and applied to totally edentulous cases receiving dental implants. However, it can be used in partially edentulous patients as well.

The technique starts with a shallow incision made approximately 10 mm from the alveolar crest and at least 15 mm distal to the site of the last implant to be placed (in the case of placing implants in totally edentulous areas). Care should be taken to ensure that the incision does not end exactly where the implants will be located. A partial thickness flap subsequently is reflected towards the crest, leaving the attached fibrous tissue over the periosteum in place, and then dissected with a scalpel to the lingual side to expose the crest of the alveolar bone. The periosteum is incised buccally and lingually next to the fibrous tissue band at the crest of the ridge. The buccal periosteum is again cut approximately 10 mm from the crest of the mandible (at the height of the first incision); the remaining fibrous tissue at the ridge crest is best removed with a rose-head bur. The implants should be placed under the crestal bone level in order not to perforate the thin remaining attached mucosa. The flap is repositioned and sutured with resorbable suture material to the buccal periosteum at its base; buccal edges of the incision are then sutured to the adjacent mucosa (Fig. 4.6a–k).

The advantages of this technique are as follows: the thickness of the mucosa is reduced to a minimal level around dental implant prosthetic components; the band of keratinized tissues is well preserved; insertion of the muscles close to the future implant site is eliminated (in the case of totally edentulous patients); primary wound closure on top of the implants is achieved, which favors healing; no additional surgical procedures are necessary to repair excessive soft issue height; more interarch space

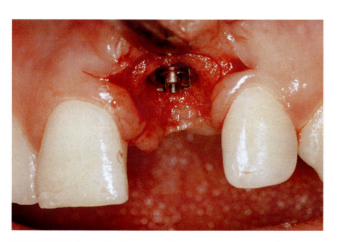

FIGURE 4.5a. Reflection of a mucoperiosteal flap through a preservative interdental papilla incision.

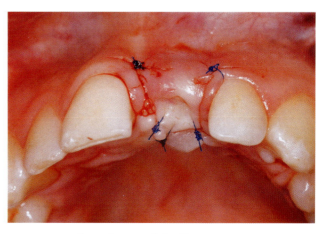

FIGURE 4.5b. Closure of the flap showing the intact interdental papillae attachment on both sides.

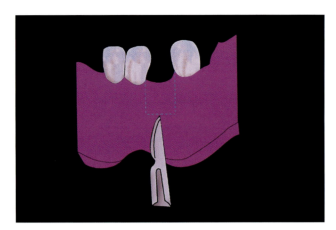

FIGURE 4.6a. An illustration showing the outline of the vestibular approach of the mucoperiosteal flap for the modified Elden & Mejchar technique for implant placement in a partially edentulous case.

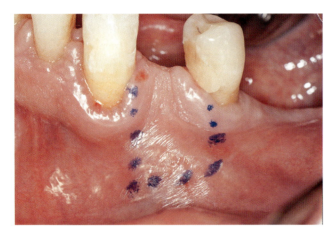

FIGURE 4.6b. The outline of the flap design marked on the soft tissue next to the space of the missing tooth.

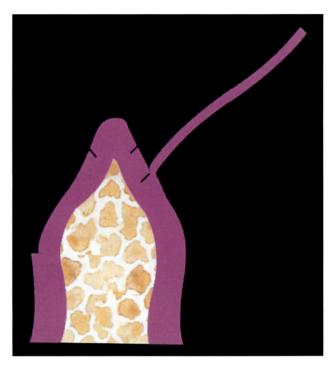

FIGURE 4.6c. An illustration showing the primary reflection of a partial thickness flap.

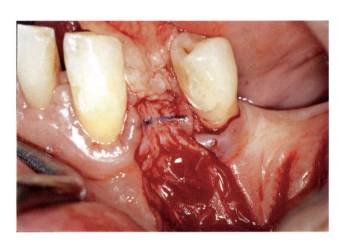

FIGURE 4.6d. The partial thickness flap reflected, with the horizontal incision marked.

will be provided for the prosthesis; and there is reduced postoperative pain for the patients because no raw areas are allowed postoperatively.

On the other hand, the procedure poses a greater risk of mucosal perforation during raising of the partial thickness flap, and possible soft tissue sloughing because the absence of the buccal periosteum reduces blood supply to the flap.

SOFT TISSUE MANAGEMENT IN IMMEDIATE IMPLANT PLACEMENT Immediate placement of dental implants in freshly extracted sites has been developed to save time and preserve the integrity of the alveolar ridge from postextraction bone resorption (Fig. 4.7).[79–87] As a consequence, primary soft tissue closure in immediate implant procedures became a vital clinical prerequisite for many authors.[88–91] Therefore, many

techniques have been used to achieve complete soft tissue closure with a satisfactory clinical outcome, either by undermining and releasing the soft tissue margins to approximate the wound edges or by applying a special surgical procedure to achieve the same goal.[61,92–97] Early exposure of immediately placed implants in fresh sockets was a common event until these new techniques offered predictable soft tissue closure results; this early exposure of dental implants might have a negative impact on osseous regenerative procedures and jeopardize implant survival rates.[91,98–102]

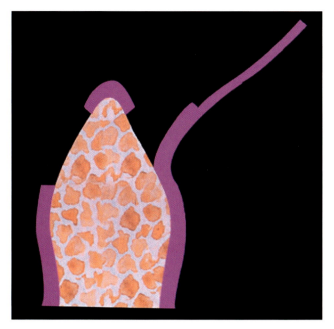

FIGURE 4.6e. An illustration showing the excision of the buccal periosteum leaving the crestal periosteum intact.

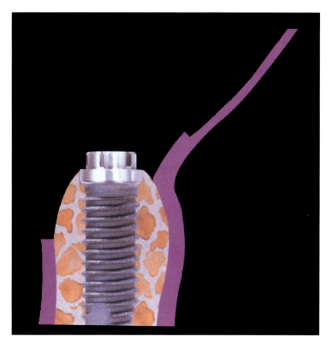

FIGURE 4.6g. An illustration showing the final placement of the implant.

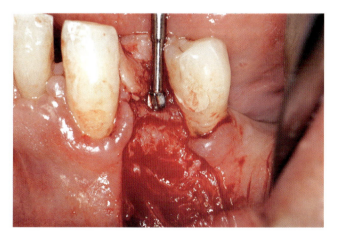

FIGURE 4.6f. The removal of the periosteum on the crest of the ridge using a large round bur and marking the osteotomy hole.

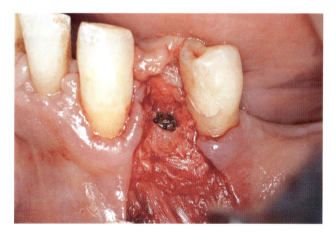

FIGURE 4.6h. View of the surgical site with the implant in place.

Adherence to the standard successful protocol for submerging dental implants that was introduced by Brånemark[103] and the need to protect the bone-grafting material from the oral environment and delay the migration of epithelial tissues into the socket walls have emphasized the importance of soft tissue closure. Yet, there is neither available scientific data to substantiate the use of one procedure over another, nor strict indications for the use of a specific surgical approach.

Complete socket closure in immediate implant placement is a technique-sensitive procedure that warrants special attention. It influences the width, position, and configuration of the attached mucosa as well as the future emergence profile.[104] The most common methods of achieving primary soft tissue closure in immediate implant placement are the palatal rotated flap, the buccal rotated flap, rehermanplasty, the pedicle island flap, and the use of guided tissue regenerative barriers.

Palatal Rotated Flap The palatal rotated flap technique was introduced by Nemkovesky et al.[105] It originally aimed at achieving primary closure on top of an immediate implant without modifying or altering the

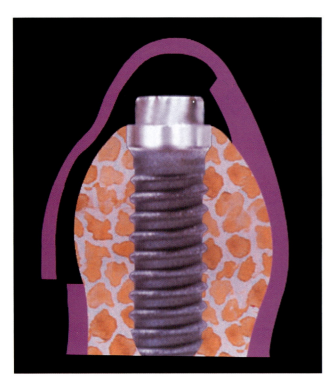

FIGURE 4.6i.   Illustration showing soft tissue closure on top of the implant.

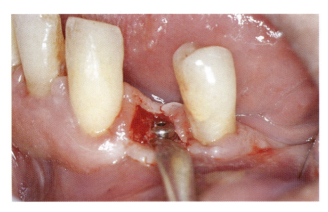

FIGURE 4.6j.   Three months after implant placement, at the time of the second-stage surgery; note the reduced gingival thickness on top of the implant head.

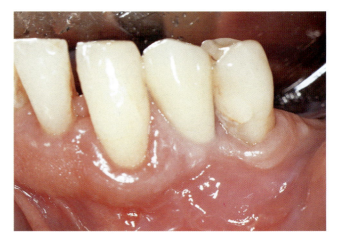

FIGURE 4.6k.   Final restoration in place.

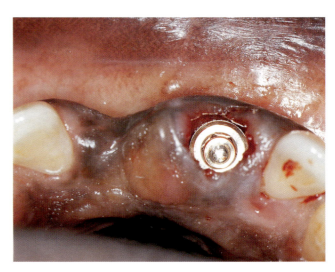

FIGURE 4.7.   A patient presented with remarkable postextraction labial bone resorption in the area of the left maxillary central incisor.

buccal contour of keratinized mucosa, which can be vital to the final aesthetic outcome of implant-supported prostheses. A palatal pedicle flap is rotated towards the buccal mucosa to cover the socket orifice (Fig. 4.8 a–e).

The technique entails an intrasulcular incision made around the maxillary tooth to be extracted and the proximal palatal aspect of the adjacent teeth; then the unsalvageable tooth is extracted atraumatically, and the implant osteotomy is prepared according to a three-dimensional aesthetic implant placement protocol. After

the implant is placed, a sharp, deep, internally beveled incision is made to delineate a full thickness palatal pedicle flap. The pedicle flap is carefully elevated from the underlying bone and rotated towards the socket orifice. Bone-grafting material is used to fill socket voids between the implant and socket walls and a GTR membrane might be placed. The pedicle flap is rotated gently using surgical pliers, then tucked and sutured to the buccal keratinized gingival margin of the socket. This procedure has shown great clinical success due to improved blood supply to the pedicle from the palatal mucosa. Therefore, the technique offers a good quality soft tissue closure while preserving the buccal integrity of the keratinized soft tissue band.

Buccal Rotated Flap   Becker and Becker[88] developed the buccal rotated flap technique to obtain a ten-

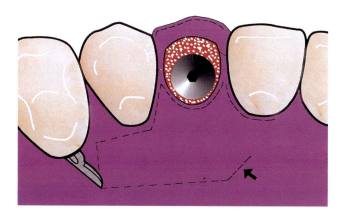

FIGURE 4.8a. An illustration showing the design of the rotated palatal flap.

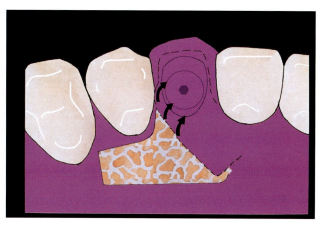

FIGURE 4.8b. Illustration showing rotation of the flap to the labial side to cover the implant site.

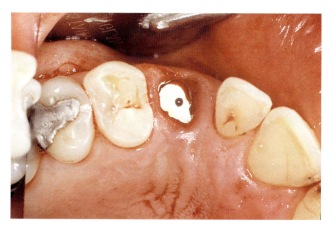

FIGURE 4.8c. An implant placed by the flapless technique, restoring missing maxillary canine.

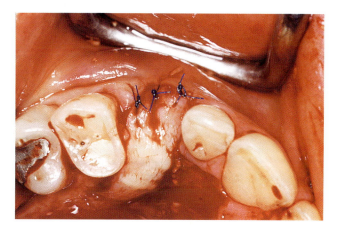

FIGURE 4.8d. A palatal rotated flap is made to cover the implant and sutured to the labial mucosa.

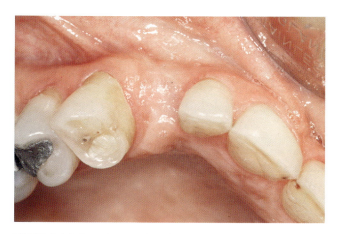

FIGURE 4.8e. Six weeks after healing.

sion-free closure on top of dental implants placed in freshly extracted sockets. The technique can achieve a complete tension-free closure without creating any mucoginigival discrepancies; however, the procedure requires advanced surgical skills in soft tissue handling. Becker and Becker originally recommended a split thickness flap from the tooth adjacent to the donor tooth to cover the exposed bone on the donor tooth itself,[88] while Novaes[106] has modified this technique by incorporating various incisions that improved the clinical outcome and reduced postoperative complications (Fig. 4.9a,b).

Novaes's technique starts by placing a vertical releasing incision at the mesial line angle of the adjacent tooth anterior to the implant site, and a second vertical releasing incision is executed at mesial line angle of the tooth lying immediately distal to the implant site. A split thickness flap is raised, starting at the first vertical incision mesially and extending to the distal line angle of the same tooth (Fig. 4.9c,d). Another deep vertical incision is then made in the periosteum, extending down to the bone to change the mode of partial thickness reflection to a full thickness reflection. All along, the elevation of the full

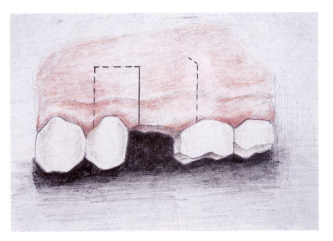

FIGURE 4.9a. An illustration showing the design of the buccal rotated flap.

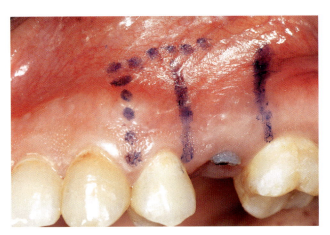

FIGURE 4.9b. A patient with an unsalvageable remaining root of the maxillary second premolar, with the outlines of the flap marked using a blue marker.

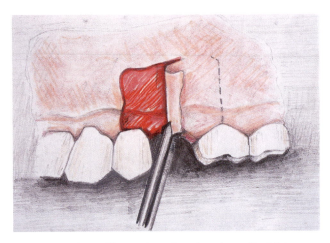

FIGURE 4.9c. Illustration showing the split thickness flap raised from the mesial side.

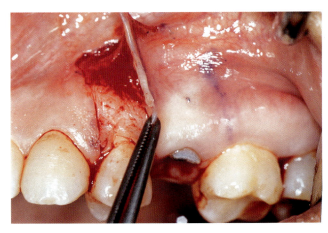

FIGURE 4.9d. Clinical view of the reflected split thickness flap.

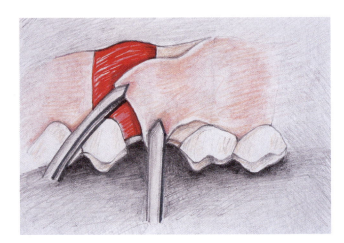

FIGURE 4.9e. An illustration showing the complete mobilization and reflection of the full thickness flap.

thickness flap is started (Fig. 4.9e–h). Any tension exerted on the flap should be avoided; a flap-relaxing incision can be made by making a small horizontal incision on the mesial aspect and most-apicovestibular part of the flap to release any possible tension. After the flap is pulled distally and coronally to cover the socket area, it is sutured to the palatal tissue (Fig. 4.9i–k). The excessive soft tissue on the distal aspect is carefully excised to facilitate closure of the distal vertical incision. The excised tissue is then used as a free gingival graft to cover the exposed periosteum over the donor tooth. Fig. 4.9l).

The main advantage of this method is that it avoids harvesting a palatal pedicled flap, which might be inconvenient for many patients (Fig. 4.9m).

Rehermanplasty Rehermanplasty is considered the most common method among clinicians for primary soft tissue closure in the oral cavity. It was originally

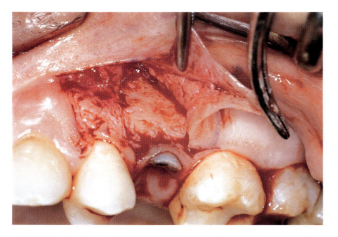

FIGURE 4.9f. Clinical view of the flap, consisting of a partial thickness segment and a full thickness segment.

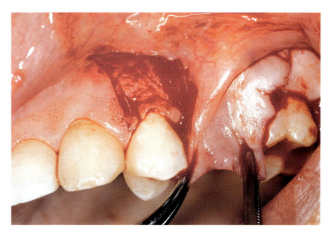

FIGURE 4.9i. View of the rotation of the buccal flap to cover the implant site.

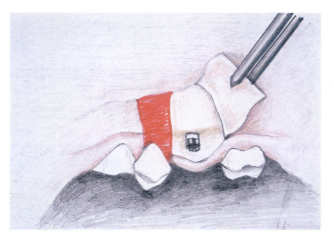

FIGURE 4.9g. Illustration showing the implant in place.

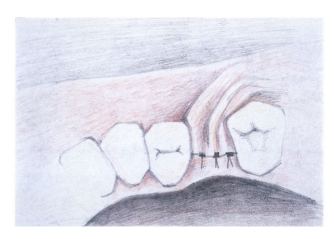

FIGURE 4.9j. Illustration showing the rotated buccal flap sutured over the implant.

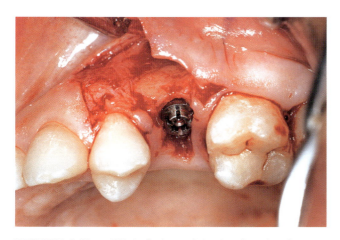

FIGURE 4.9h. Clinical view of the implant in place.

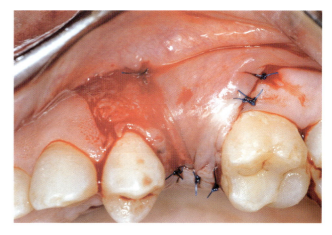

FIGURE 4.9k. The rotated buccal flap is sutured.

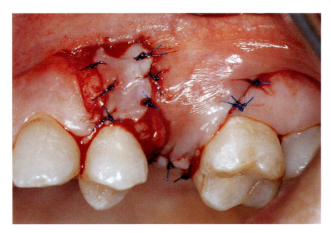

FIGURE 4.9l. A free gingival graft excised from the excessive soft tissue distally covers the exposed periosteum.

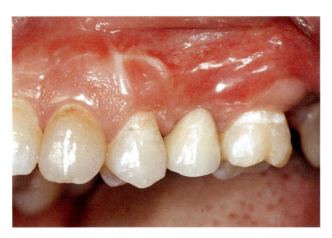

FIGURE 4.9m. The final restoration in place.

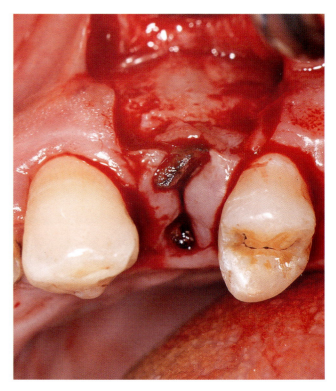

FIGURE 4.10a. A mucoperiosteal flap designed for immediate implant placement.

developed to close oroantral fistulae.[107,108] It is currently used successfully to achieve primary soft tissue closure in immediate implant placement cases. This method entails raising a full thickness mucoperiosteal flap through two vertical parallel incisions that are made along both sides of the extraction socket and extended vestibularly (Fig. 4.10a). The flap is then reflected and extended farther vestibularly (Fig. 4.10b). A periosteal slitting incision is then made horizontally at the base of the flap, after which multiple incisions in the periosteum can be made to lengthen and release the flap if required. The flap is then released and extended to cover the socket and sutured to the palatal or lingual mucosa.

This method provides an excellent predictable socket seal but is not satisfactory from an aesthetic point of view because the attached buccal mucosa shifts from its original position to the crest of the ridge, thus losing its continuity (Fig. 4.10c). Nevertheless, this mucogingival discontinuity can be corrected during second-stage

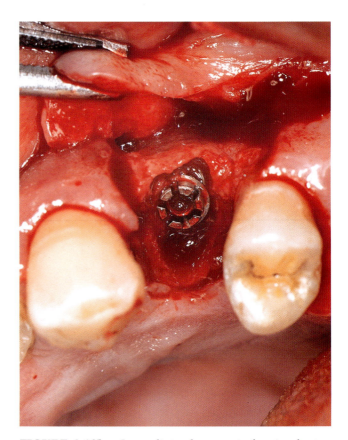

FIGURE 4.10b. Immediate placement of an implant.

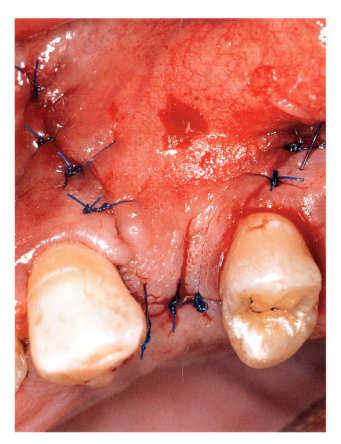

FIGURE 4.10c. Complete soft tissue closure.

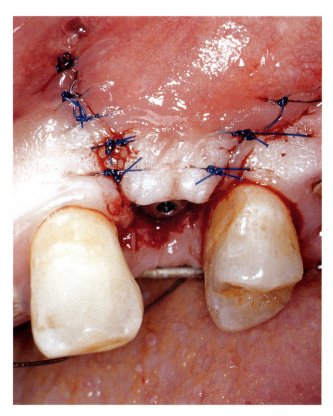

FIGURE 4.10d. Apically repositioned flap at the second-stage surgery with the healing abutment in place.

surgery. This can be achieved by apical repositioning the keratinized tissues from the crest of the ridge to the labial side, thus restoring soft tissue integrity (Fig. 4.10d,e).

Pedicle Island Flap

The pedicle island flap is used to achieve soft tissue closure in immediate implant placement procedures. It offers a predictable socket closure and achieves an excellent aesthetic postoperative result: in this technique the attached buccal mucosa is not altered or repositioned, and therefore the mucogingival integrity is kept intact.

After the implant is placed in the fresh extraction socket (Fig. 4.11a,b), two parallel horizontal incisions are made in the vestibular mucosa, creating a tongue-like extension (Fig. 4.11c,d). The base of the mucosal extension is placed posterior or distal to the socket opening. The flap is made approximately 20 mm long and as wide as the socket width. The surface of the mucosal extension is thereafter deepithelialized, except for the apical portion that corresponds to the surface of the extraction socket (Fig. 4.11e,f). A subperiosteal tunnel connecting the marginal keratinized mucosa is then made, buccal to the extraction socket and the corresponding site in the vestibule (Fig. 4.11g,h). The flap extension is subsequently pulled through the tunnel until the epithelialized apex of the flap covers the socket and then sutured to the attached free gingiva from the palatal side of the socket (Fig. 4.11i,j). Finally, the vestibular wound is approximated and sutured (Fig. 4.11k,l).

The base of the mucosal extension exhibits a rich blood supply, which enhances the predictability of the technique.[109] It also provides proper tissue seal on top of the socket (Fig. 4.11m). However, the delicate nature of the mobile soft tissue making up the mucosal extension may create difficulty in clinical handling. The mucosa can easily be torn or lacerated, especially during the dissection or deepithelialization of the tongue-like mucosal extension. The color difference between the extension and the surrounding attached mucosa makes it a distinct island of vestibular tissues to be identified and excised at the second-stage surgery (Fig. 411n,o).

Guided Tissue Regeneration

Soft tissue management to achieve primary closure in immediate implant placement can sometimes be a difficult clinical task that has an increased potential postoperative risk of complications. Using guided tissue regenerative (GTR) barriers to close the socket orifice has been claimed to help eliminate the need for soft tissue closure.

The technique involves a horizontal incision extending along the marginal gingiva of two teeth adjacent to the

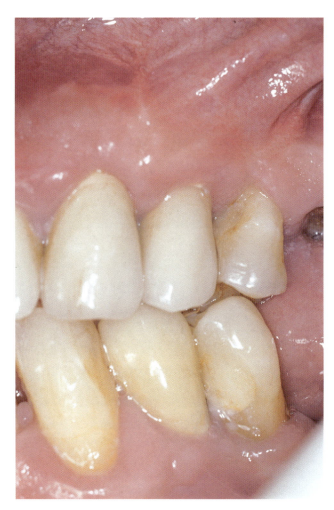

FIGURE 4.10e. View of the final restoration cemented in place.

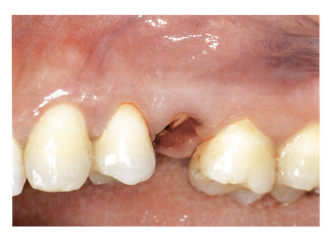

FIGURE 4.11a. A patient with a remaining root of a maxillary second premolar.

extraction site from both buccal and lingual sides.[110] The mucoperiosteal flap is then reflected without vertical releasing incisions, and the implant is placed (the socket

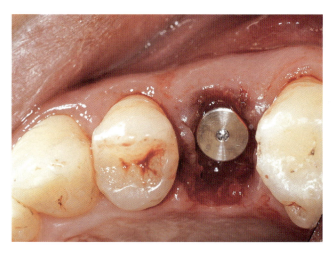

FIGURE 4.11b. Flapless placement of an implant into the fresh extraction socket.

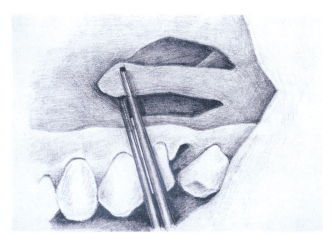

FIGURE 4.11c. Illustration showing the tongue-like extension dissected from the vestibular mucosa.

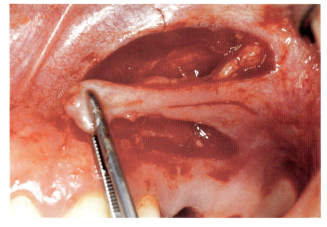

FIGURE 4.11d. The tongue-like extension on the buccal side after being released.

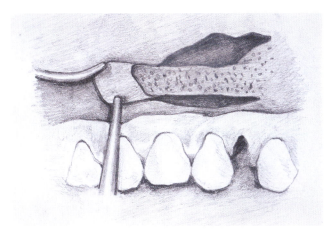

FIGURE 4.11e. Illustration showing the partial deep-ithelialization of the extension except for its apical part.

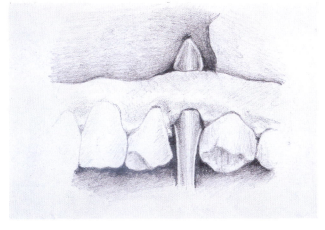

FIGURE 4.11h. An illustration showing the subperiosteal tunnel created.

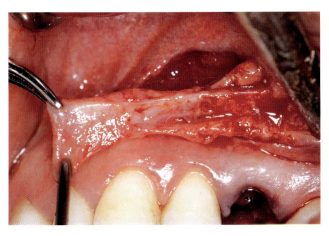

FIGURE 4.11f. The mucosal extension is partially deepithelialized.

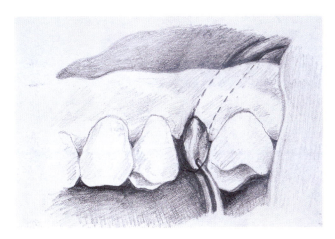

FIGURE 4.11i. An illustration showing the mucosal extension being tucked underneath the tunnel to cover the socket.

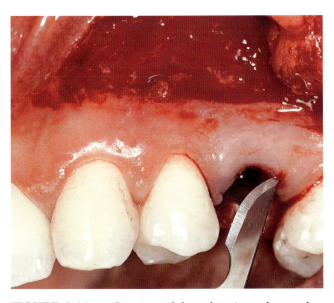

FIGURE 4.11g. Creation of the subperiosteal tunnel using a scalpel.

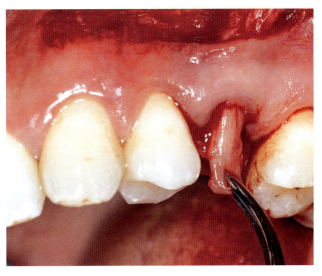

FIGURE 4.11j. The mucosal extension appearing from the tunnel after being pulled.

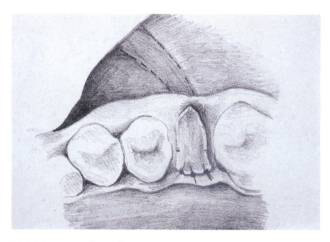

FIGURE 4.11k. Illustration showing the mucosal extension sutured to the palatal free gingival margins of the socket.

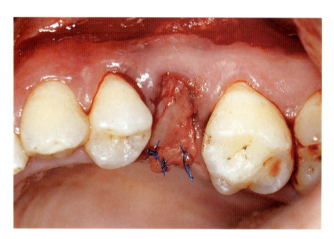

FIGURE 4.11l. View of the socket closed.

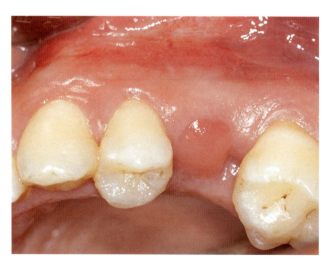

FIGURE 4.11m. Four weeks after surgery, showing favorable healing; note the color distinction between the tongue-like extension and the surrounding attached tissue that gives the shape of an island.

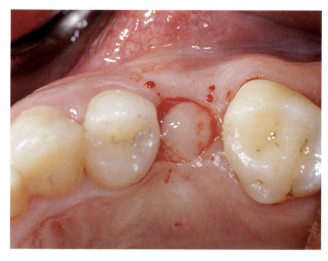

FIGURE 4.11n. Second-stage surgery using the punch technique, only removing the soft tissue pedicle island.

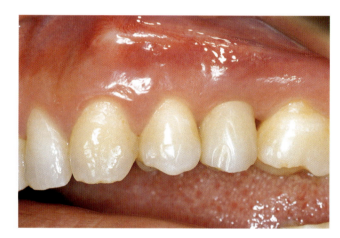

FIGURE 4.11o. The final restoration in place. Note the continuity of the keratinized tissue band.

voids may be grafted). A homologous cortical bone membrane (Lambone™, Pacific Coast Tissue Bank, Los Angeles, California, U.S.A.) is tucked above the implant head and underneath the flap at least 5–6 mm under the mucoperiosteum, buccally and lingually; this type of membrane is preferred due to its high biocompatibility.

The membrane should fit precisely to the bone from each side. The flap is then returned to its place with the membrane secured in place, and sutured. The central area of the membrane is left exposed, allowing tissues to migrate over it and, given ample of time, to heal completely.

Using GTR instead of the soft tissue techniques to close freshly extracted sites can be questionable, as this technique is considered highly susceptible to infection because the hostile environment of the oral cavity favors bacterial population on top of or underneath the membrane. Furthermore, the possible formation of granulation tissue underneath the membrane can lead to its loosening, which can compromise the predictability of the bone-grafting procedure or the osseointegration.

Socket Seal Template Technique   The use of soft tissue closure procedures in immediate implant cases can be tedious and increases the risk of postoperative complications; in most cases it can result in postoperative discomfort for patients. In an attempt to provide a treatment alternative to the (sometimes) complicated soft tissue closure procedures, a new technique is introduced to achieve the same purpose. The new socket seal template technique aims at isolating the implant and the bone graft in immediate implant placement from the oral environment. This technique is particularly recommended for use when a flapless immediate implant placement technique is performed.[111,112] A custom-made acrylic template is fabricated and placed on top of the implant and the bone graft, thus sealing the socket. Using this method may reduce the likelihood of soft tissue complications. The procedure can be of great benefit to patients possessing a thin scalloped tissue biotype, where soft tissue shrinkage can be a common postoperative event. Lastly, but most importantly, it preserves both the soft and hard tissue architecture.[113,114]

The technique entails a thorough and precise clinical performance with utmost regard for the nature of the existing oral tissues at the time of implant placement. The procedure involves atraumatic extraction of the unsalvageable tooth to ensure intact undamaged socket walls. After debridement of the socket walls is performed, the implant is placed according to the aesthetic placement protocol. The voids between the implant and the socket walls (if they exist) are filled with the bone-grafting material of choice. Using maximum implant size is recommended to ensure a greater primary anchorage of the implant (Fig. 4.12a). A tailored collagen pack (Cola Tape, Centerpulse, Dental Division, Carlsbad, Califor-

nia) is placed on top of the graft in order to prevent loss of the graft particles during clinical handling; then a temporary abutment (Centerpulse, Dental Division, Carlsbad, California) is connected to the implant and trimmed to the required height.

Self-cure acrylic resin in its rubbery stage of curing is introduced to the socket and packed around the temporary abutment. It is withdrawn along with the temporary abutment just before final curing occurs to prevent tissue exposure to the heat emitted from the polymerization reaction (Fig. 4.12b). Once polymerization is completed extraorally, the template is trimmed and polished to remove the excess material and to snugly fit into the socket (Fig. 4.12c), then secured in place with the temporary abutment

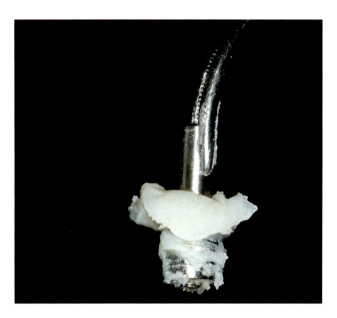

FIGURE 4.12b.   Self-cure acrylic resin attached to the temporary abutment before trimming.

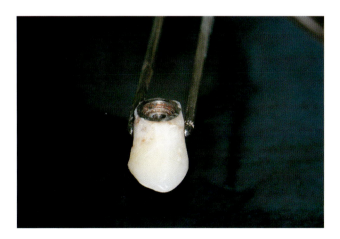

FIGURE 4.12c.   The temporary abutment ready for insertion after trimming and polishing the excess resin material.

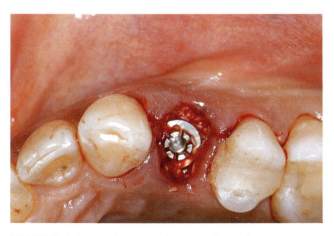

FIGURE 4.12a.   An immediate implant placement with the socket voids filled with bone grafting material.

connecting screw. An antibiotic and antianaerobic ointment may be applied on its fitting surface before it is secured in place. The seated template should be at approximately the same level as or slightly below the marginal gingiva. It is possible to remove the template at any later time to clean it and put it back in place.

After the recommended healing period for the implant and the bone graft has elapsed, a natural-looking emergence profile around the implant site that attains the same cervical dimension as the original missing tooth is replicated (Fig. 4.12d). The need for emergence profile development using a provisional prosthesis or wide healing abutments at this time is eliminated; therefore, this procedure is considered to be time saving. Impressions are made using transfer copings at the time of the removal of the template in order to obtain the exact profile before the soft tissue collapses, and a provisional restoration is fabricated and fitted to the temporary abutment after the acrylic resin material is removed (Fig. 4.12e).

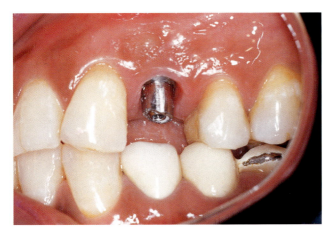

FIGURE 4.12d. The final abutment in place. Note the natural soft tissue profile devolved.

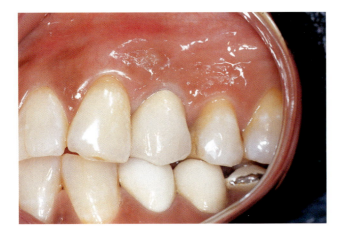

FIGURE 4.12e. The case finally restored.

Using the socket seal template technique has several advantages. It may prevent the apical migration of the gingival epithelium into the socket and the bone graft. Additionally, it favors tissue healing from the periodontal ligament site,[115] as periodontal ligament cells are capable of migrating only for short distances.[116,117]

In immediate implant placement, the regular soft tissue manipulations around dental implants, especially in thin scalloped tissue biotypes, can result in a greater amount of soft tissue shrinkage.[76,118] The possibility of soft tissue shrinkage around the socket seal template during clinical manipulation is much less likely to occur.[119,120]

The use of GBR (guided bone regenerative) membranes or GTR (guided tissue regenerative) membranes in conjunction with implant placement has been highly controversial. It has not been confirmed that there is conclusive evidence of improved survival of bone grafts when GTR membranes are used, especially in small osseous defects around implants.[93,97,121] Therefore, the application of a barrier membrane may not be mandatory in any immediate implant placement procedures. Others have strictly recommended the use of a barrier membrane to help stabilize both the blood clot and bone graft material[122] before epithelial migration occurs. It has been claimed that the socket seal template can provide a function that is similar to GBR membranes.

Advantages of the socket seal template technique may be summarized as follows:

- It protects the bone grafting material around the dental implant.
- It eliminates soft tissue trauma.
- It minimizes patient discomfort postoperatively.
- It isolates the implant from the hostile environment of the oral cavity.
- It supports the marginal surrounding soft tissues and prevents postextraction bone resorption.
- It provides an exact replica of the emergence profile of the missing tooth for the future implant-supported prosthesis.
- It reduces the treatment time as it eliminates the time required for doing a second-stage surgery.
- It reduces treatment cost.
- It satisfies the patient's aesthetics.
- If an immediate loading protocol is the treatment of choice, it can allow an immediate provisional prosthesis to be fabricated on top of the template.

The socket seal template technique should be limited to patients with excellent oral hygiene, areas that allow a placement of a minimum 13 mm long implant, a mechanically well stabilized implant in the socket, and small osseous defects around the dental implant that do not exceed 1 mm circumferentially.

FLAPLESS TECHNIQUE FOR IMPLANT PLACE-MENT The flapless, immediate placement technique is utilized to maintain the natural soft tissue contours, preserve alveolar ridge integrity, and avoid additional soft tissue trauma by raising a mucoperiosteal flap. Preservation of the delicate vascular network adjacent to implant receptor sites may be an important factor in maintaining facial bone height and aesthetics. In edentulous regions where the vascular network is compromised by tooth loss, the associated periosteum and soft tissues may serve as primary blood sources for the area. Some authors[111,112,123] have reported the use of a flapless approach for immediate and delayed dental implant placement in the alveolar ridge. A study[124] evaluated the clinical success of osseointegration achieved with nine immediate implants placed without incisions in fresh extraction sites, and without any guided bone regenerative membranes being used; the only allowed grafting material to fill the socket gaps was autogenous bone chips harvested from the drilling procedure. Interestingly, the results showed high clinical success without soft tissue primary closure. The study was based on the fact that there is no absolute necessity for either bone augmentation or primary flap closure when placing implants in freshly extracted sites.[124] In other words, the absolute need for soft tissue closure for dental implants placed in fresh extracted sites has not yet been proven.

Another study[125] used nonsubmerged implants in healed sites and exposed the alveolar bone with a mucosal punch; the authors stated that placing an implant without raising a mucoperiosteal flap reduces surgical morbidity and postoperative bone resorption. Furthermore, it stabilizes the papillary height after surgery and has an increased patient acceptance.

In the case of immediate implant placement, the clinical procedure for the flapless placement technique starts with an atraumatic extraction of the unsalvageable teeth. Drilling is then performed through a surgical template with the use of a buccally placed guiding finger, to avoid perforating the labial plate of bone. Autogenous bone chips are collected from the drill flutes and packed back into the surgical site around the implant fixture to fill any existing gaps. Finally, the wound edges are approximated and may be sutured.

This approach is utilized to avoid soft tissue complications, including postoperative recession. It also helps to simplify the implant surgery for both the patient and clinician, as achieving primary closure with immediate implant placement sometimes may be considered a difficult task. In the delayed implant placement protocol where gum punching is used to expose the bone for the drilling procedure and implant placement, the flapless technique may help achieve acceptable aesthetic results and reduce postoperative complications (Fig. 4.13a–c).

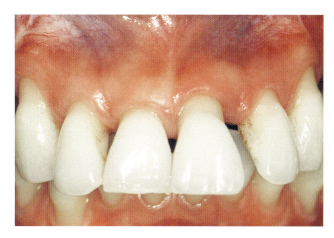

FIGURE 4.13a. Preoperative view of four unsalvageable maxillary anterior teeth to be replaced with dental implants; note the thin scalloped tissue biotype of the patient that warrants flapless implant placement.

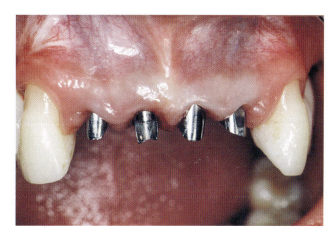

FIGURE 4.13b. Postoperative view showing the abutments connected; the interimplant papillae are preserved.

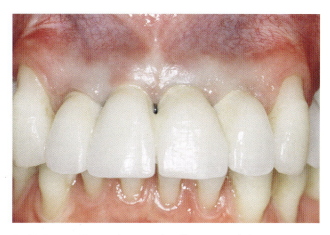

FIGURE 4.13c. The case finally restored showing intact peri-implant architecture.

Factors that are considered to be detrimental to this treatment modality include lack of direct visibility, difficulty in assessing any labial osseous defects at the time of implant placement, the absolute necessity of using axial tomography or a CT scan preoperatively to evaluate the osseous topography, the limited ability to augment implant sites due to lack of visibility, and the potential loss of almost 4 mm of keratinized tissue at the time of implant placement due to gum punching (in case of the delayed implant placement protocol). In addition, the potential contamination of the implant surface by the soft tissue surrounding the surgical site might complicate the overall prognosis. A conservative palatal flap may be reflected during implant placement, which can reveal the condition of the labial plate of bone; it can be viewed through the palatal side at a 45 degree angle to the occlusal plane. This modified palatal approach adds more predictability by helping to detect any labial osseous defect before implant placement.

In conclusion, the flapless approach is still a blind surgical procedure that should be approached with caution and performed only by skillful experienced clinicians.[123]

MUCOPERIOSTEAL FLAP CLOSURE IN CRITICAL CONDITIONS   Osseous grafting of the alveolar ridge is always required to increase the height or width of a deficient alveolar ridge. Therefore, primary soft tissue closure on top of the graft is a major concern and should be permitted to protect the graft because it favors uninterrupted healing and contributes positively to the graft success. Furthermore, failure to achieve tension-free closure of the mucoperiosteal flap might negatively affect graft survival or implant osseointegration.[67,126,127] Therefore, complete tension-free closure should be achieved to accomplish an uneventful wound healing. Excessive clinical manipulations performed to achieve tension-free primary closure can lead to soft tissue trauma, which negatively affects the quantity and quality of regenerated bone.[127] Consequently, many atraumatic surgical approaches to soft tissue coverage over grafted sites have been developed over the past twenty years.[35,99,128]

Fugazzotto,[127] detailed the surgical management and closure of mucoperiosteal flaps on top of grafted sites with GBR techniques. This surgical protocol of soft tissue closure is considered the most reliable method of achieving primary closure on top of grafted sites, and it helped many practitioners to solve many clinical problems. The broad outlines of the clinical procedures are as follows: (1) extend the vertical incisions from the crest of the ridge to the vestibular mucosa, (2) undermine the flap with another two horizontally placed vestibular incisions, and (3) make a deep periosteal slitting incision at the base of the flap.

The surgical procedure for grafting an intraoral deficient osseous site commences with a crestal incision placed slightly to the palatal or lingual side and extending at least one tooth mesial and distal to the site to be regenerated. This is followed by two vertical releasing incisions extending to the buccal vestibule (Fig. 4.14a–f). Another

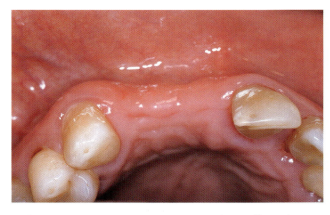

FIGURE 4.14a.   Preoperative view of maxillary alveolar bone resorption.

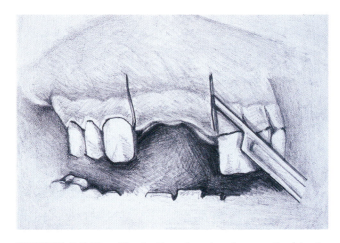

FIGURE 4.14b.   Illustration showing two vertical incisions made.

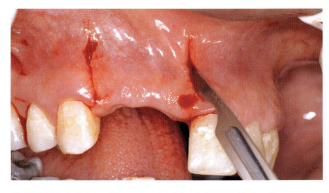

FIGURE 4.14c.   Two vertical incisions clinically.

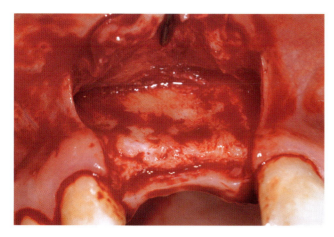

FIGURE 4.14d. The mucoperiosteal flap reflected revealing the nature of the defect.

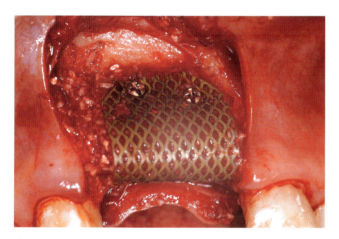

FIGURE 4.14e. Titanium mesh carrying bone-grafting material is used to treat the osseous defect (note the change of the alveolar ridge size).

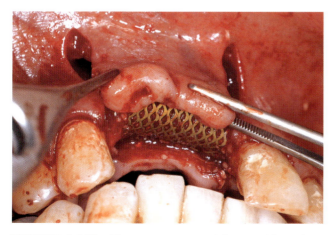

FIGURE 4.14f. The mucoperiosteal flap could not be stretched to achieve edge-to-edge closure.

Two horizontal releasing incisions are made, starting from the most apical extent of the vertical releasing incisions and extending 3–4 mm anteriorly and posteriorly in the buccal vestibule (Fig. 4.14g,h). After a full thickness flap is raised, a horizontal incision at the deepest part of the base of the flap is made on the periosteum to release the flap and allow for further stretching (Fig. 4.14i,j). The incisions can be repeated in other areas of the periosteum until a sufficient flap lengthening is acquired, so that both edges of the flap can be approximated without tension (Fig. 4.14k,l). These surgical manipulations will consequently alter the mucogingival continuity (Fig.

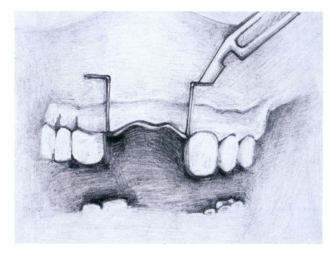

FIGURE 4.14g. An illustration showing the two vestibular horizontal incisions.

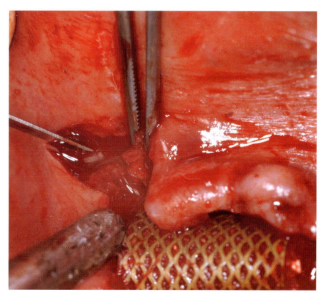

FIGURE 4.14h. The two horizontal incisions intraorally.

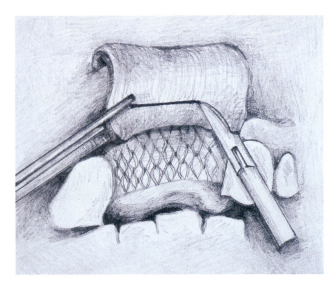

FIGURE 4.14i. An illustration showing a deep horizontal periosteal slitting incision.

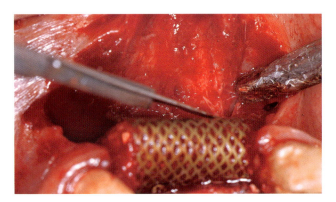

FIGURE 4.14j. Deep horizontal slitting incision made intraorally.

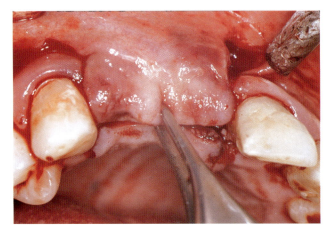

FIGURE 4.14k. The flap is mobilized and stretched to achieve tension-free primary edge-to-edge closure.

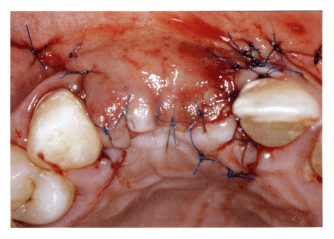

FIGURE 4.14l. The flap sutured.

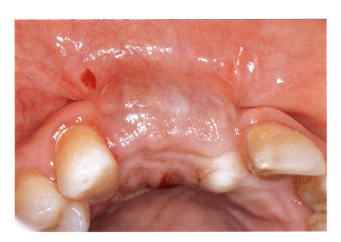

FIGURE 4.14m. One month after healing occurs; note the discontinuity of the attached mucosa.

4.14m), which can be corrected later with another repositioning corrective surgery (Fig. 4.14n).

Other attempts[128,129] to allow tension-free soft tissue closure on top of grafted sites while maintaining the position of the labial mucogingival junction at its original level have been introduced. A palatal flap approach is used to overcome this clinical situation: the palatal flap is elongated through a split thickness dissection; as a result of the split thickness incision, a connective tissue extension is reflected with the palatal flap over the crest of the ridge. The flap with the connective tissue pedicle is then slid in a labial direction to cover the augmented area without interrupting the continuity of the labial keratinized tissue band. The palatal connective tissue extension is then sutured to the labial soft tissue margin. However, this procedure has limitations when thin palatal tissue exists, which complicates the partial thickness reflection procedure. Additionally, the

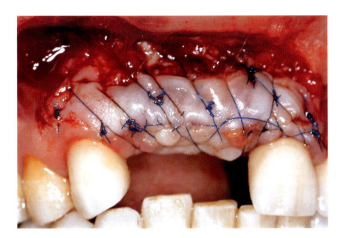

FIGURE 4.14n. Free gingival graft combined with vestibuloplasty is performed to improve the attached mucosa condition. This step is taken to improve the clinical results for the second-stage surgery.

amount of tissue gained from the palatal flap lengthening might not always be sufficient.

Soft Tissue Management at the Time of Abutment Connection

The form and quality of the soft tissue adjoining the implant components are vital prerequisites for ensuring a natural-looking implant-supported restoration. The nature of the alveolar mucosa mandates an excellent second-stage surgery protocol to help regain the missing biological emergence profile and related soft tissue contours. Due to an increasing demand for natural-looking implant-supported restorations by both clinicians and patients, new surgical techniques have been introduced, especially those pertaining to the aesthetic zone.

Soft tissue manipulation at the time of abutment connection is conceptual. There are no strict recommendations that can be applied to the protocol of the second-stage surgery. The techniques vary according to the future vision, experience, and preference of the clinician. In selecting from the many techniques available, the clinician should consider all those techniques that aim at modifying the soft tissue contours and simulating natural appearance. Also to be chosen are those techniques in which the adjacent papillae are manipulated to accommodate the future implant-supported restoration in a natural-looking manner.

The second-stage surgery in the aesthetic zone is not only performed to expose the implant interface for executing restorative procedures, but also to create a healthy marginal attached mucosa around the implant components.[103] All the basic intraoperative precautions, including the selection of an optimal flap design, that ensure sufficient blood supply and allow for better access and visibility must be strictly observed to maintain uneventful healing. The use of cosmetic incisions is highly recommended in the second-stage surgery[130] because they are beveled toward the center of the flap at a 45 degree angle, thereby minimizing the chances of postoperative soft tissue scarring, while at the same time favoring healing.

Two basic surgical protocols are used to expose the implant head at the second-stage surgery. The first is conservative and is basically performed by reflecting a mucoperiosteal flap next to the implant to be restored. The second is excisional: the soft tissue on top of the implant head is excised to reveal the cover screw. This second protocol can be called the soft tissue punching technique.

RULES OF SECOND-STAGE SURGERY

To improve the soft tissue status around the implant prosthetic components at the time of second-stage surgery, some clinical guidelines for reducing postoperative complications and maximizing the aesthetic outcome can be helpful. These "rules" are not obligatory, because the decision to use them will ultimately be the clinician's to make. Rather, they are clinical recommendations that can be applied separately in different clinical situations or together in a single surgery. By using these guidelines as a clinical reference, the clinician can obtain satisfactory aesthetic results. The goal of creating natural-looking soft tissue profiles around dental implants may be achieved by adhering to the following "rules": bulking keratinized or connective tissues facially, scalloping the keratinized tissues, limiting the incision to the keratinized tissues, preserving intact interproximal papillae, and using connective tissue grafts in conjunction with second-stage surgery.

Bulking Keratinized or Connective Tissues Facially

This rule aims at the displacement of soft tissues from the palatal to the labial aspect, which in turn leads to soft tissue bulking and overprofiling around the prosthetic components. Technically speaking, this procedure can be described as a reverse Rehermanplasty (Fig. 4.15a,b).

Increasing the amount of keratinized tissues on the facial aspect of the prosthetic components is necessary to develop the future biological width and to compensate for any postoperative soft tissue remodeling or gingival recession. A longitudinal study conducted by Bengazi

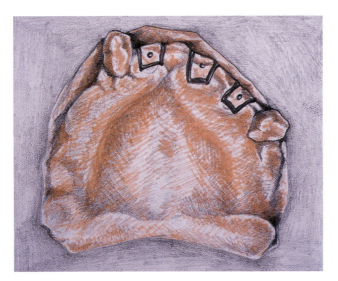

FIGURE 4.15a. Sketch on a study model showing the incision design at the second-stage surgery that moves the palatal keratinized mucosa to the labial side.

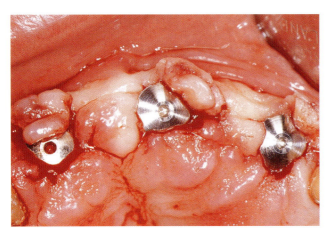

FIGURE 4.15b. Clinical application of bulking the keratinized mucosa labially around healing abutments.

et al. that measured the alterations in the position of peri-implant soft tissue margin on partial and full arch implant-supported prostheses after the second-stage surgery.[119] The study revealed a gingival recession of 0.4 mm on the labial aspect of implant-supported prostheses in the maxilla after six months, and 0.7 mm after twenty-four months in nongrafted sites. It was proposed that the recession of the peri-implant soft tissue margin may be mainly the result of a remodeling of the soft tissue in order to establish an appropriate biological dimension. Another confirming study conducted by Grunder[120] evaluated the soft tissue stability around ten single-tooth implants. All cases were treated with guided bone regen-

eration and connective tissue grafting. One year after prosthesis insertion, 0.6 mm of soft tissue shrinkage was recorded on the buccal side of the implant-supported prosthesis.

It is not inconceivable that soft tissue shrinkage is expected around implant-supported dental restorations in the first six months following abutment connection. These findings favor the concept of bulking the keratinized mucosa as much as possible on the labial aspect to compensate for any soft issue shrinkage. It also supports the use of a provisional prosthesis for six months after abutment connection, until a stable gingival margin is obtained.

Following complete maturation of the soft tissue after the second-stage surgery, when the gingival margins have reached a stable level, any excessive soft tissue that exceeds the adjacent natural contour can be trimmed off and removed. At the time of the second-stage surgery, not only should keratinized tissues be bulked around the abutment, but also connective tissue grafts can be used to treat minor osseous defects around dental implants or to provide a root-eminence-like profile. A connective tissue graft is placed underneath the mucoperiosteal flap and secured with resorbable sutures to improve the soft tissue profile (Fig. 4.16a,b,c).

Scalloping the Keratinized Tissues

To ensure proper soft tissue adaptation to the circular shape of the prosthetic components a C-shaped incision is made palatal to the implant head, with the convexity of the C directed buccally, during the second-stage surgery. At the end of the C scallop, two small (1–2 mm) vertical relieving incisions are made to allow for flap

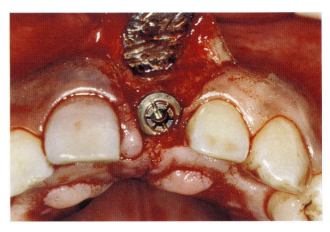

FIG 4.16a. A clinical view showing a minor alveolar ridge deficiency around an implant replacing a maxillary left central incisor.

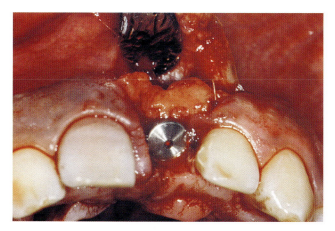

FIGURE. 4.16b. Connective tissue graft is used at the time of the second-stage surgery to bulk the soft tissue profile.

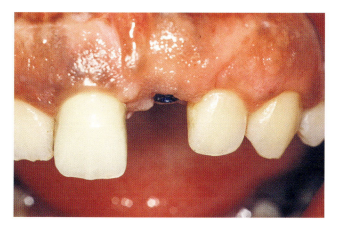

FIGURE 4.16c. Clinical view six weeks after abutment connection showing an improved peri-implant soft tissue contour imitating the bulging root shape, which gives a natural appearance to the implant-supported prosthesis.

mobility. The flap is then raised, the abutment is connected, and the flap is pushed backward until the scallop is adapted to embrace the buccal aspect of the abutment collar (Fig. 4.17a,b). This method ensures tighter adaptation of the soft tissue to the abutment, thus reducing the tendency for developing a dead space and minimizing any possible soft tissue marginal discrepancy around the abutment.

Hertel et al.[103] described another procedure that serves a similar purpose. They called it the cervical folding technique. This technique achieves an intimate flap abutment adaptation around the prosthetic components as well (Fig. 4.18).

Limiting the Incision to the Keratinized Tissues

It is the author's experience that extending the vertical relieving incisions to the vestibular tissues should be avoided at the second-stage surgery in order to avoid any possible postoperative soft tissue scarring (Fig. 4.19).

Hertel et al.[103] advocated a second-stage surgery design that provides incisions only in the keratinized mucosa and maintains a proper amount of keratinized tissue around the implant collar (see Fig. 4.20a,b). They described the placement of an incision on the crest of the ridge. This incision is followed by bisection of the attached mucosa with two small proximal vertical incisions around the implant to release the tension on the flap.

Preserving Intact Papillae

Preserving the interproximal papillae in the second-stage surgery or keeping them intact is a strict recommendation for preventing further drop down or recession of the adjacent marginal soft tissues, as recommended in cosmetic periodontal surgeries.[131–134] Therefore, the decision not to displace the papillae from their original location is conceivable and will contribute positively to the stability of the soft tissue margins. This approach averts postoperative soft tissue shrinkage around natural dentition as well as the implant prosthetic components (see Fig. 4.21). Preserving the interproximal papillae might also reduce soft tissue trauma during the surgery.

Using Connective Tissue Grafts in Conjunction with Second-Stage Surgery

Many authors have used connective tissue grafts at the time of the second-stage surgery to treat minor soft tissue deficiencies or simulate a rootlike bulging around the neck of the implant-supported prosthesis.[135–137] Abrams[135] introduced an interesting method for augmenting minor edentulous alveolar defects. The technique involved stripping the epithelium from a palatal connective tissue pedicle and rolling it under the buccal mucosa; this procedure has shown high clinical predictability for improving the alveolar ridge topography at the defective area. Scharf and Tarnow[138] introduced a modification of Abrams' technique. A "trap-door" approach is used to reflect and preserve the epithelium that overlies the connective tissue pedicle; the epithelial pedicle is used to cover the donor site, thus eliminating any raw area at the donor site.

The technique requires reflecting an epithelial flap with a connective tissue extension or pedicle from the palate and moving it to the site to be augmented labially. Two

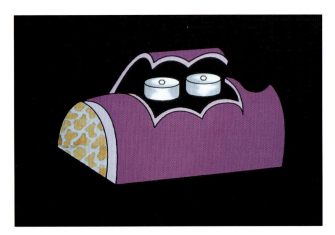

FIGURE 4.17a. Illustration showing the scalloped incision design around healing collars.

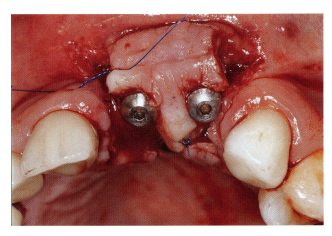

FIGURE 4.17b. Clinical view of the scalloping of keratinized mucosa around healing collars.

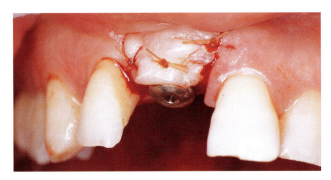

FIGURE 4.18. Tying the keratinized tissues around the abutment to help proper adaptation.

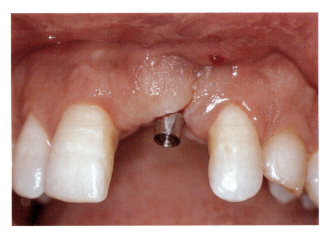

FIGURE 4.19. Example of soft tissue scarring, due to extending the incision line to the vestibular mucosa during second-stage surgery.

full thickness vertical parallel releasing incisions are made from the crest of the ridge toward the palate to outline the pedicle, preserving the papillae in both sides of the defect

as much as possible. The length of the incisions is dependent on the length of connective tissue required. The two vertical incisions are joined with a shallow horizontal incision along the crest of the ridge to be a starting point for the partial thickness reflection of the epithelial flap. Once the epithelial flap is reflected, an incision is made along the connective tissue pedicle, down to the bone. The connective tissue pedicle is now bounded laterally by the two vertical incisions made initially for the epithelial pedicle and apically at its base by another horizontal incision to separate it. The connective tissue pedicle is then reflected in an apicocoronal direction. A pouch between the buccal mucosa and the alveolar ridge is made. The connective tissue pedicle is then rolled into the buccal pouch and secured with sutures. The epithelial pedicle is replaced over the bone and secured.(Fig. 4.22a–h).

The use of the modified roll flap technique for soft tissue enhancement therapy prior to implant placement increased the amount of connective tissue at the defective area, which in turn improved peri-implant soft tissue contours and reduced patient discomfort to a great extent by preventing denudation of the palatal bone.

The author[139] introduced the use of the modified roll flap technique at the time of the second-stage surgery. It is proposed that healing abutments can provide support for the rolled connective tissue pedicle, which in turn improves the final soft tissue profile and simulates the rootlike eminence. Using the modified roll flap at the time of the second-stage surgery is indicated only when minor defects exist; larger defects mandate surgical corrective procedures before starting the implant therapy (see Fig. 4.23a–f).

Soft Tissue Punching

Soft tissue punching is another surgical alternative for exposing the implant cover screw at the second-stage

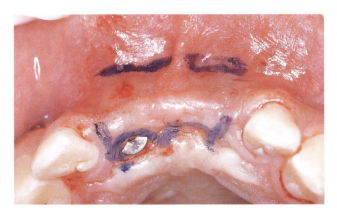

FIGURE 4.20a. Incision design for nonresorbable membrane removal during the second-stage surgery to avoid extending the two vertical incisions to the vestibular tissues.

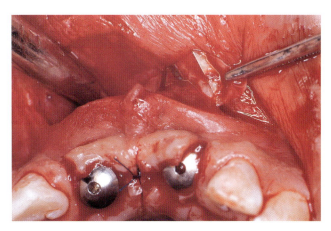

FIGURE 4.20b. Removal of the nonresorbable membrane from the buccal vestibule; note the limited vertical incision.

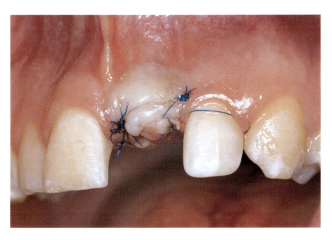

FIGURE 4.21. Preservation of the interdental papillae in second-stage surgery to avoid postoperative shrinkage. Note the amount of keratinized tissues being bulked on the labial side.

surgery. The technique entails excising a circular area of the keratinized mucosa on top of the implant cover screw, which makes the technique excisional in nature. The technique has limited indications; it is only indicated when a wide and stable keratinized band is present, and it can be applied safely in the posterior zone where aesthetics are not of prime concern.

The use of the soft tissue punching procedure can offer some advantages. It is a simplified clinical technique, less traumatic to the tissues, and does not require an extensive surgical inventory to be applied, as it can be performed with a scalpel, a gum-punching tool, or a diamond bur.

On a precautionary note, punching of soft tissues has its drawbacks. Imperfect positioning of the tissue punch may jeopardize the labial peri-implant contour integrity,

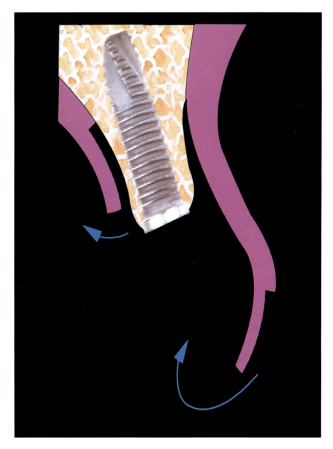

FIGURE 4.22a. Illustration showing the modified roll flap in second-stage surgery.

and the attendant subsequent loss of almost 3–4 mm of keratinized tissue limits its application in the aesthetic zone. Furthermore, tissue punching sometimes involves guesswork in locating the implant head unless the original surgical template is used; the implant cover screw can

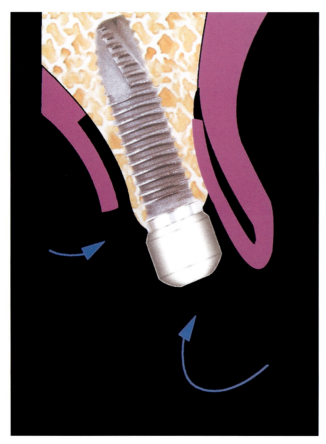

FIGURE 4.22b. Illustration showing rolling of the palatal flap extension underneath the labial flap.

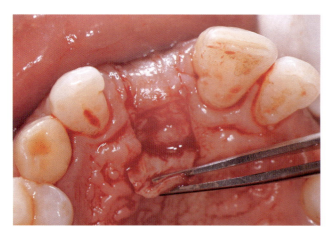

FIGURE 4.22c. Two vertical incisions with the reflection of the partial thickness palatal flap.

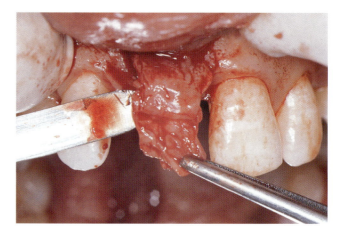

FIGURE 4.22d. The connective tissue pedicle attached to the labial mucosa after dissection.

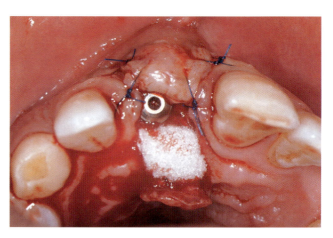

FIGURE 4.22e. Suturing of the flap after the connective tissue pedicle has been rolled underneath the labial soft tissues.

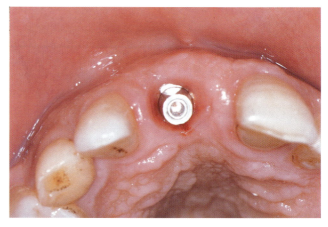

FIGURE 4.22f. Postoperative view showing a remarkable improvement of the labial contour.

be located by searching the area with a sharp probe until it catches the cover screw (sound of metal scratching can be heard). When an implant is placed below the bone

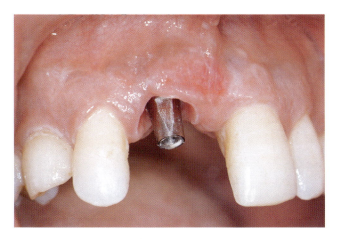

FIGURE 4.22g. The final abutment in place.

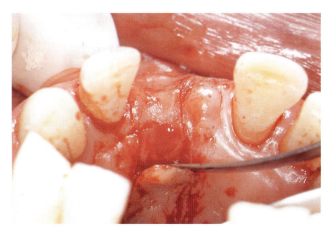

FIGURE 4.23b. The two vertical incisions made along the reflection of the palatal partial thickness flap.

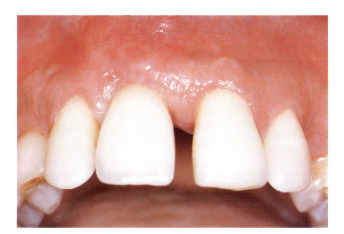

FIGURE 4.22h. The case finally restored.

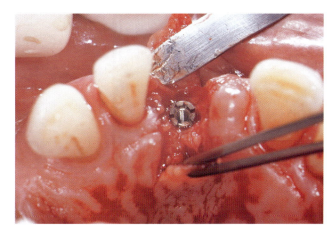

FIGURE 4.23c. Mobilization of the connective tissue pedicle.

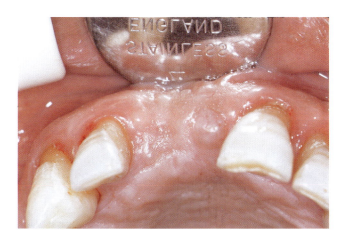

FIGURE 4.23a. Preoperative view showing minor labial defect.

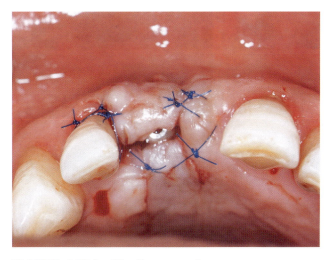

FIGURE 4.23d. The flap sutured.

crest level, bone contouring may be recommended, as it creates a funnel-like shape in the bone to accommodate the flaring of the prosthetic component, but with the

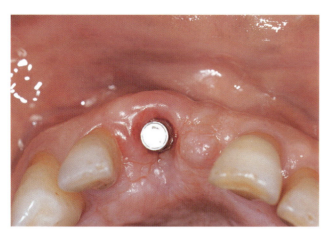

FIGURE 4.23e. The labial contour is improved and the final abutment connected.

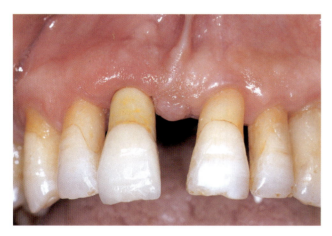

FIGURE 4.23f. The case finally restored.

punching technique, it may be difficult to apply particular bone-contouring tools. Care should be exercised not to injure the surrounding soft tissue while removing any excess bone on top of the implant head.

STM POSTABUTMENT CONNECTION

Manipulating the soft issue after the prosthetic components are connected to the implant fixture can be called peri-implant tissue refining and profiling. After the second-stage surgery, when complete tissue healing has occurred, the peri-implant soft tissues can be reshaped or augmented to attain a satisfactory aesthetic outcome, to overcome some resultant tissue defects, and/or to treat some tissue deformity (e.g., dimples, ditched-in tissues, grooves); therefore, this stage of implant therapy can be called plastic implant soft tissue surgery.

Miller was the first to introduce mucogingival surgery, or periodontal plastic surgery.[140] Such surgical procedures are used to correct or eliminate anatomic, developmental, and/or traumatic deformities of the gingiva and alveolar mucosa. These surgical procedures are currently applied in conjunction with implant therapy to help achieve an enhanced peri-implant soft tissue appearance. Using plastic soft tissue surgery around dental implants eliminated the use of soft-tissue-colored prosthetic devices that were used to mask soft tissue defects.

Corrective procedures may involve one or more of the following treatment options: onlay grafting; inlay grafting; connective tissue pouch procedures; and gingival recontouring procedures, which involve (a) modifying and expanding the gingival margin with the use of a provisional restoration, (b) plastic soft tissue grafting to treat soft tissue grooves or deficiencies, (c) sculpting the excessive soft tissues, and (d) contouring of the marginal gingiva.

Onlay Grafting

Onlay soft tissue grafting techniques, including their clinical modifications, are becoming popular methods among clinicians for treating peri-implant soft tissue defects. The techniques have been extensively described in the literature.[32,141–144] These techniques originally aimed at increasing the width of keratinized tissues, treating mucogingival defects, and arresting gingival recession around natural teeth.[145] Onlay soft tissue grafting may be performed prior to implant placement (Fig. 4.24) or after connection of the final abutment, to improve the integrity of soft tissue contours, stabilize soft tissue margins, and treat minor deficiencies.[146] Moreover, it can be used to mask undesirable soft tissue pigmentation, such as amalgam tattoos (Fig. 4.25a,b).

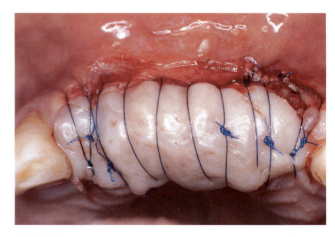

FIGURE 4.24. Onlay graft to treat an alveolar ridge defect.

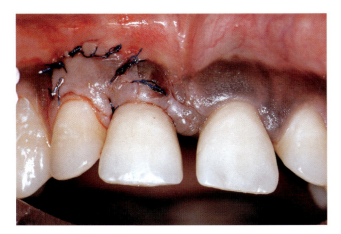

FIGURE 4.25a. Onlay graft has been performed to treat a keratinized tissue discontinuity.

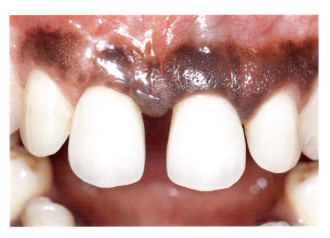

FIGURE 4.25b. Postoperative view showing the healing of the graft and the recovered keratinized tissue continuity.

Adherence to the basic intraoperative principles of soft tissue grafting, such as determining the amount of soft tissue required to cover the defect, the clinical condition of the recipient site, and the availability of donor tissues, detecting the location of any anatomical landmark in the area of grafting, and assessing the patient's oral hygiene condition can be considered important clinical steps that favor the final clinical results.[7] The final soft tissue dimensions gained from any onlay grafting procedure are directly related to the thickness of the graft used and the amount of tissue that survives the grafting procedure.[23] But it is generally accepted that a thin graft is used for increasing the zone of attached tissues, whereas a thick graft is recommended for ridge augmentation procedures. If greater tissue height is required from an onlay soft tissue grafting procedure, the procedure may be repeated after a two- to three-month interval until an optimal tissue contour is achieved (Fig. 4.26a–d).

The procedure entails two surgical sites: the recipient site, and the donor site. The recipient site is prepared by an incision that starts at the distal end of the defect with the blade held parallel to the alveolar process; then the blade is drawn in a mesial direction to the end of the defect. Another horizontal incision (equal in length to the first) is made just below the mucogingival junction. The residual band of keratinized tissues will be removed to allow for epithelial denudation, which can be achieved with a scalpel or high-speed bur. A sharp dissection is performed apically to separate the alveolar mucosa and muscle fibers from the periosteum, and it is preferred to overextend the periosteal bed to compensate for any expected future shrinkage of the graft. The graft size is then determined using a tin foil cut to the exact size of the recipient bed.

The donor site (usually the palate) is prepared by making a beveled incision, starting along the occlusal aspect of the palate and continuing apically, while lifting and sepa-

rating the graft as it moves. A tissue forceps is used to retract the graft distally until it is finally separated. The graft should be trimmed to remove any fatty, glandular tissues, or tissue irregularities, which might inhibit the graft-take. After the graft is prepared, it is adapted and fitted to the underlying periosteum and sutured. Five minutes pressure with saline-wetted gauze will permit fibrin clot formation and prevent postoperative bleeding. Coverage of the grafted area with rubber dam material (to prevent the sutures from adhering to the dressing) followed by a surgical dressing on top may be recommended.[147] Coverage of the raw area of the donor site relieves patient's postoperative discomfort; it can be achieved by fitting a previously fabricated acrylic template to the palate.

The clinical drawbacks and complications encountered with onlay grafts include the color and texture mismatch between the graft and the surrounding tissues (tire patch appearance), the difficulty of graft adaptation to the recipient site, graft mobility due to hematoma formation, graft shrinkage (approximately 30%) from its original size after healing is complete,[148] and the difficulty of achieving proper adherence of the graft to titanium abutments, which has caused some clinicians to abandon this grafting procedure after the abutment connection.[149]

A recent development in onlay grafting procedures is the introduction of the acellular dermal matrix (Alloderm, Lifecore Biomedical). Grafting with autogenous tissue or freeze-dried skin can be an accepted method for increasing and/or restoring the width of attached gingiva. The method was originally used to treat burn patients. When used as a gingival graft, it possessed major potential advantages over the traditional onlay grafts, including improved color and contour match to the original tissues, elimination of donor site surgery, and unlimited availability.[150]

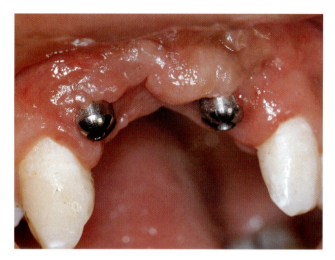

FIGURE 4.26a. Severe soft tissue defect due to several failed bone grafting attempts.

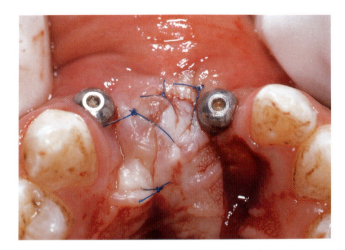

FIGURE 4.26b. Bilateral pedicle graft from the palate to enhance the quantity and quality of tissue on the crest of the alveolar ridge.

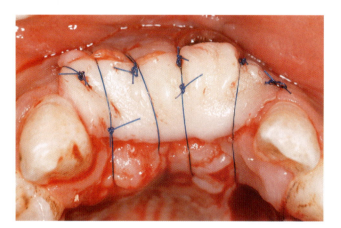

FIGURE 4.26c. Onlay graft is utilized with vestibuloplasty to improve the labial contour and vestibular status.

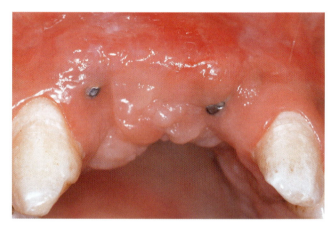

FIGURE 4.26d. The case six weeks after healing. Note the improvement in the pontic area as well as in the sulcus depth.

Inlay Grafting

Langer and Calagna[33, 137] were the first to outline the clinical indications and description for the use of subepithelial connective tissue grafts to cover a denuded root surface or to augment the alveolar ridge for aesthetic reasons. The technique was later modified and improved by others.[137,140] The technique of using inlay grafting showed success and predictability in treating one-, two-, and three-dimensional soft tissue defects around natural teeth and dental implants. Interestingly, 2–6 mm of root coverage has been documented in cases where subepithelial grafts are used to treat denuded root surfaces.[137] This technique is now used routinely by many clinicians to enhance soft tissue profile with implant-supported dental restorations.

Connective tissue grafts are applied clinically in two different forms: (1) a graft composed solely of connective tissue or (2) a graft composed of connective tissue that has an epithelial rim (a composite graft). The connective tissue grafts are used for aesthetic ridge augmentation procedures, while the composite grafts are used for treating denuded root surfaces and masking gingival discoloration around dental implants.

The inlay grafts have an advantage over the onlay grafts because they combine the characters of the soft tissue autograft and the pedicle flap procedure.[152] This combination doubles the blood supply to the graft, thus increasing its chances of survival; also, inlay grafts attain the same color and texture of the tissues surrounding the recipient site after healing has occurred. Grayish gingival discoloration around dental implants is a result of the metallic reflection (of the prosthetic components) through a thin mucosa; it affects the aesthetic outcome of the implant-supported prostheses negatively, especially in patients with a high smile line. Connective tissue inlay grafts can treat the condition successfully, as the inlay graft masks gingival discoloration by increasing the thickness of the peri-implant soft tissues (Fig. 4.27a–d). In this particular case, the graft should be proximally extended farther from the implant site to compensate for the reduced blood supply to the graft, thereby allowing peripheral anastomosis from the adjacent tissues.

The procedure involves two main clinical steps: (1) preparation of the recipient site and (2) harvesting the graft. A horizontal intrasulcular incision is made on the marginal gingiva with the scalpel angle parallel to the tooth long axis; another two vertical incisions are made

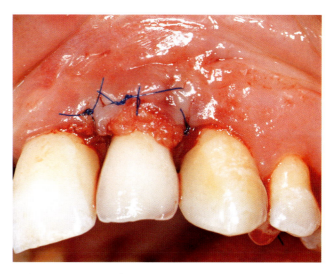

FIGURE 4.27c. The connective tissue graft secured in place underneath the labial tissue. Note that no vertical incisions are made.

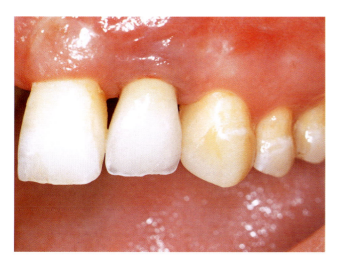

FIGURE 4.27a. Preoperative view showing soft tissue grayish discoloration related to an implant-supported restoration replacing the maxillary left lateral incisor.

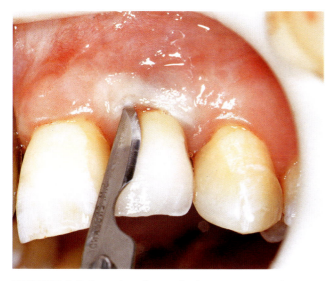

FIGURE 4.27b. One-line sulcular incision made at the recipient site with the scalpel parallel to the long axis of the teeth.

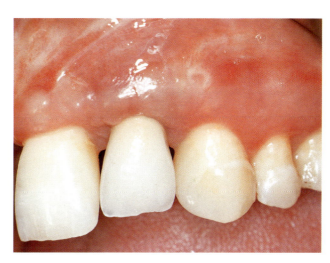

FIGURE 4.27d. Six weeks after healing, showing clinically improved soft tissue that masks the metallic collar of the abutment.

to facilitate mucoperiosteal flap release. A partial thickness flap is then raised by blunt dissection until it reaches the vestibule. Care must be exercised not to perforate the flap during dissection and thus jeopardize the overall blood supply.

The connective tissue graft can be harvested from the palate or from the tuberosity. A straight, horizontal incision parallel to the alveolar ridge starts posteriorly at approximately 5–6 mm from the free gingival margin and is extended anteriorly. A second, more coronally positioned, parallel incision is made approximately 3 mm from the free gingival margin and is continued to the same distance as the first incision. Then two small vertical incisions are made mesially and distally to connect the two horizontal incisions. Another horizontal incision is made at the apical border of the graft to completely separate the graft from the underlying bone. This will finally provide a 2–3 mm wide connective tissue wedge with an epithelial rim. Finally, the palate is sutured with continuous basting sutures.

The graft is then trimmed and introduced into the recipient site, drawn underneath the partial thickness flap, and secured with a sling suture to the labial mucosa. In aesthetically demanding areas where only increased tissue height is required, no vertical relaxing incisions should be made at the recipient site, to avoid any possibility of future scar tissue formation.

Connective Tissue Pouch Procedures

The connective tissue pouch procedure is another clinical modification for using connective tissue grafts; it is used to correct confined minor ridge deficiencies, where the color and surface characteristics of the area after grafting should not differ from the original tissue character (Fig. 4.28a–e).[22,23,136,137]

The procedure is indicated when the alveolar defect is not large in size and does not jeopardize the function of the

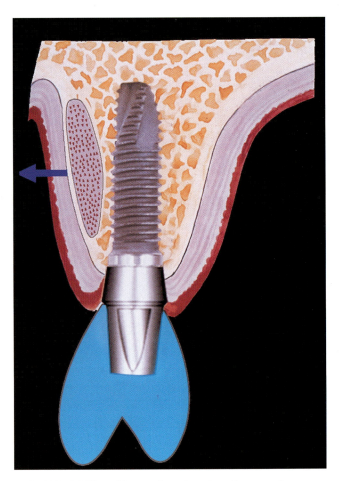

FIGURE 4.28b. Illustration showing the use of connective tissue graft to improve the labial contour.

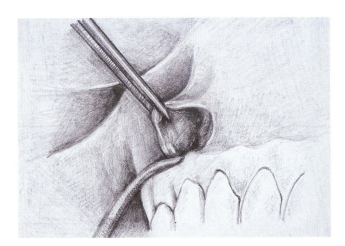

FIGURE 4.28c. Illustration showing the pouch created in the labial mucosa with a one-line vertical incision.

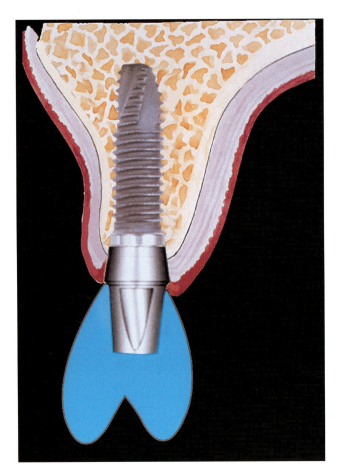

FIGURE 4.28a. Illustration showing minor labial defect related to the implant.

implant. However, the long-term clinical results of the graft are still questionable. Initially, this procedure exhibits remarkable postoperative results, but graft shrinkage as a

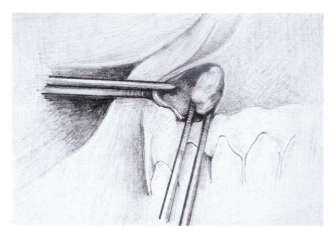

FIGURE 4.28d. Illustration showing the connective tissue graft being introduced to the pouch.

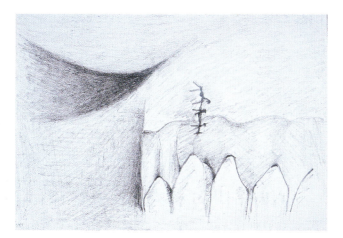

FIGURE 4.28e. Illustration showing the final closure.

result of postoperative tissue remodeling has a tendency to occur over time. The procedure can also be called a "closed connective tissue grafting procedure" because the graft is totally embedded under the soft tissues, thus providing more predictable graft survival.

The procedure involves making a supraperiosteal pouch at the deficient area; a one-line vertical incision, extending apically and bypassing the deformity through the attached gingiva and the mucogingival junction, is made. Blunt dissection is used to extend the pouch. The maxillary tuberosity and the palate are readily accessible donor sites for harvesting the connective tissue graft to repair the alveolar defect. A 2 to 3 mm thick connective tissue graft is carefully dissected, deepithelialized, introduced to the pouch, and placed underneath the flap. The graft is then stabilized with resorbable sutures. A suture is first passed through the base of the pouch to the end of the graft, then another suture is made in the middle of the graft, which helps stabilize the graft to the underlying periosteum; the pouch is then closed with interrupted sutures (Fig. 4.29a–f).

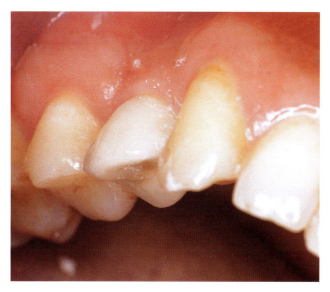

FIGURE 4.29a. Clinical view showing labial defect around an implant-supported restoration replacing a missing maxillary first premolar.

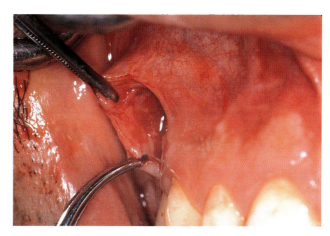

FIGURE 4.29b. The pouch is created through a one-line vertical incision.

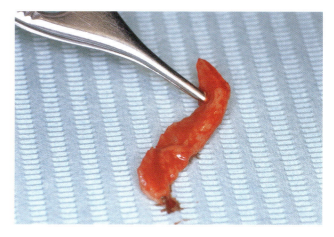

FIGURE 4.29c. The connective tissue graft is harvested.

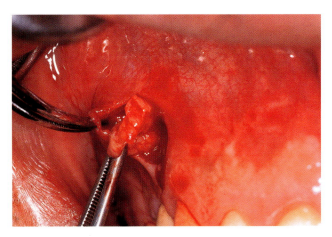

FIGURE 4.29d. The connective tissue graft is introduced into the pouch.

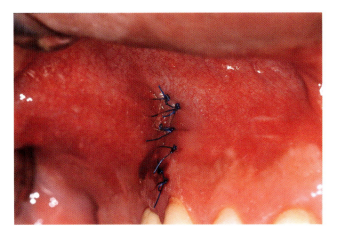

FIGURE 4.29e. The pouch is closed and sutured.

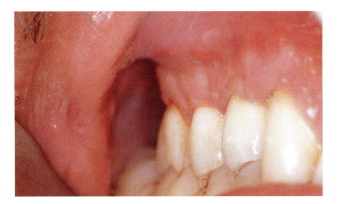

FIGURE 4.29f. Postoperative view showing improvement of labial contour.

In extremely compromised defects where bone grafts are not indicated, a connective tissue graft can be used in combination with another onlay graft.[153] The connective tissue graft is placed underneath the defect to restore tis-

sue volume, while the epithelial graft can stabilize mucosal margins and increase the width of the attached mucosa. Combining two types of grafting procedures increases soft tissue height and stability. However, postoperative soft tissue remodeling remains an issue for concern (Fig. 4.30a–f).

Gingival Recontouring Techniques

Gingival recontouring techniques[154] are plastic surgical procedures used to reshape or refine peri-implant soft tissues, and they are usually performed after the implant is restored. The techniques require a favorable keratinized tissue condition, in terms of quality and quantity. The techniques include cosmetic laser resurfacing, electrosur-

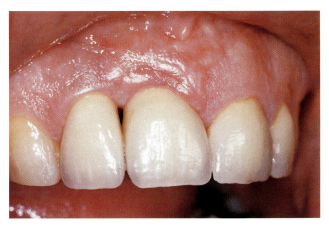

FIGURE 4.30a. A remarkable loss of the interimplant papilla between two implant-supported crowns replacing the maxillary right central and lateral incisors.

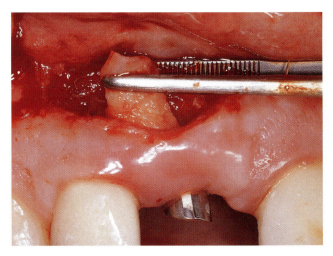

FIGURE 4.30b. A connective tissue graft is being introduced and tucked underneath the defect from a vestibular approach in order to provoke a downward movement of the interimplant papilla.

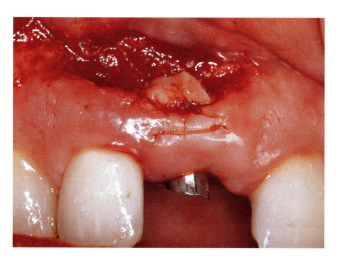

FIGURE 4.30c. The connective tissue graft is secured and sutured to the underlying periosteum.

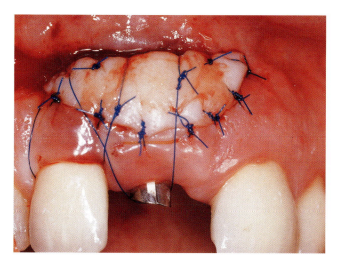

FIGURE 4.30d. An onlay graft is used to compensate for the downward movement of the vestibular tissue as well as to stabilize its new position.

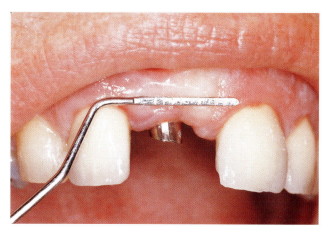

FIGURE 4.30e. Six weeks postoperative healing, showing an improvement of the interimplant papilla height.

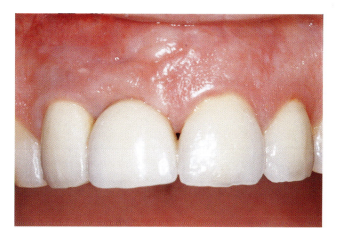

FIGURE 4.30f. Final crown inserted.

gical sculpturing, gingivoplasty, and the use of provisional restorations.

COSMETIC LASER RESURFACING[130] Peri-implant soft tissue irregularities sometimes occur after the completion of the implant therapy as a result of multiple surgical procedures or due to uneventful soft tissue healing. They can be soft tissue dimples or irregularities that affect the aesthetic outcome of the implant-supported restoration negatively, especially if the patient possesses a high smile line. It clinically appears as soft tissue nodes or white elevated scar lines in the peri-implant soft tissue area. Cosmetic laser soft tissue resurfacing is widely used by plastic surgeons because it has been shown to control the depth of tissue removal better than any other traditional method, it allows for precise tissue trimming, it offers a bloodless field, and it emits less heat generation to the underlying tissues than do rotary instruments.

ELECTROSURGICAL SCULPTURING Electrosurgery can be used to remove the excess bulky gingival contours or smoothen tissue scars, as is done in laser resurfacing. Tissue warming due to the heat emitted from the electrodes sometimes delays healing. This method should be applied with caution because there is an increased risk of implant failure if the electrode contacts the implant surface.

GINGIVOPLASTY Minor plastic surgical procedures known as gingivoplasty can be used to treat undesirable aesthetic gingival contours, provided a sufficient amount of keratinized tissue is present. It is usually limited to patients with the thick flat tissue biotype, where

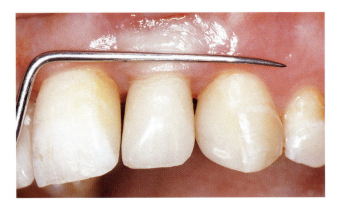

FIGURE 4.31a. Excess keratinized mucosa around an implant-supported restoration after the insertion of the final prosthesis.

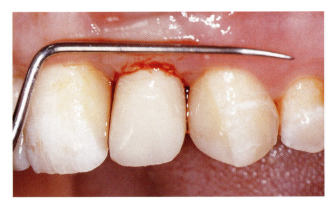

FIGURE 4.31b. The excess gingival tissues were excised with a scalpel.

the condition of the soft tissue can withstand further surgical manipulations. It is used when final maturation of the soft tissue around the implant-supported restoration has occurred. The procedure entails removal of the excessive facial gingival tissues using either a sharp scalpel (Fig. 4.31a,b) or a high-speed diamond bur (Fig. 4.32).

USE OF PROVISIONAL RESTORATIONS An implant-supported provisional restoration is considered an important tool for reshaping and profiling the peri-implant soft tissues without performing any surgical intervention after the second-stage surgery is completed and soft tissue is healed. It is considered the most important factor responsible for a natural appearance of implant-supported restorations. It stimulates peri-implant tissues to attain the same configuration and dimensions as missing original natural soft tissue contours. After the peri-implant tissues are duplicated on the working cast, envisioned, and carved to the optimal

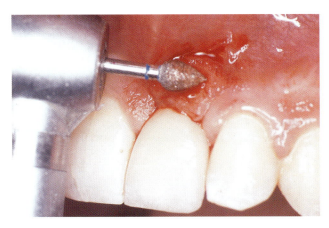

FIGURE 4.32. Trimming of keratinized tissue dimple with a diamond bur.

desired configuration, a provisional restoration is fabricated accordingly and transferred to the implant site. The provisional prosthesis is then seated. Digital pressure is exerted to compress the peri-implant tissue in an outward labial direction. Temporary blanching of the soft tissue occurs as a result of the pressure, resulting in changing of the soft tissue contours to the future final implant-supported restoration dimension.[154]

THE REAL PAPILLAE

Creating an aesthetic implant-supported restoration in the oral cavity depends to a great extent on the presence of healthy peri-implant soft issue architecture.[155] The presence of the interproximal papillae around implant-supported restorations allows symmetrical soft tissue margins and a state of harmony between natural and dental implant components.[31] The slightest change in the level of the interproximal papillae around dental implants due to pathologic reasons or poor soft tissue handling during implant treatment can lead to major aesthetic and phonetic complications.

After tooth extraction, the thin adjacent alveolar bone (interradicular bone) starts to undergo a rapid process of resorption, probably due to the thin nature of the alveolar bone (which allows faster resorption), reduced blood supply to the crest of the interradicular bone due to the tooth extraction procedure, the possible direct exposure of the interradicular bone to oral bacteria as a result of tooth extraction, and most importantly, the absence of the Sharpey's fibers that stimulate continuous bone remodeling and thus maintain healthy marginal levels. As a result of tooth extraction, the interdental papilla remodels in a sloping fashion from the palatal to the more apical facial osseous plate, and becomes depressed in comparison with the healthy adjacent marginal tissue.[156] Unfortunately the lost interdental papilla is not capable of self-regeneration to regain its original dimensions.[157] This complicates the overall clinical prognosis and mandates special reconstructive procedures.

The greatest challenge today in implant and periodontal plastic surgery is the reconstruction of lost or incomplete interproximal papillae. Many clinical efforts have attempted to reconstruct the missing interproximal papillae by using guided tissue regenerative procedures,[158] augmenting procedures,[159] free gingival grafts,[160] coronally positioned flaps,[161] pedicle grafts,[151] and pontic development techniques.[1] Unfortunately, no single technique for papilla regeneration offers predictable long-term clinical success.

To assess and classify the different clinical conditions of the interdental papillae, Nordland et al. have classified the clinical condition of the interdental papillae according to their marginal level.[162] They subdivided the interdental papillae into three classes (Fig. 4.33a–d):

- *Class I.* Tip of the interdental papilla lies between the interdental contact point and the most coronal

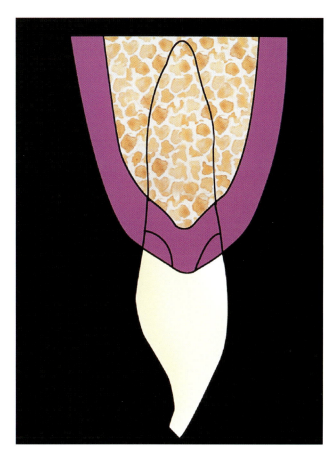

FIGURE 4.33b. Class II Nordland classification.

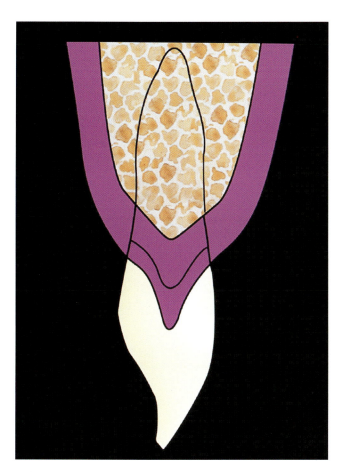

FIGURE 4.33a. Class I Nordland classification.

extent of the interproximal CEJ (space is present, but interproximal CEJ is not visible).
- *Class II.* Tip of the interdental papilla lies at or apical to the interproximal CEJ (interproximal CEJ visible).
- *Class III.* Tip of the interdental papilla lies level with or apical to the facial CEJ.

Tarnow et al.[163] developed a useful classification for clinically identifying the predictability of the presence of interdental papillae. They concluded that when the measurement from the contact point of the natural tooth to the crest of the bone was 5 mm or less, the papilla was present almost 100% of the time; when the distance was 6 mm, the papilla was present 56% of the time; and when the distance was 7 mm or more, the papilla was present in only 27% of the time or less (Fig. 4.34).

Salama et al.[164] proposed another interesting classification that furnished a prognostic classification system for the peri-implant papillae. Their three classes are based on the available interproximal height of bone (IHB) in relation to the prognosis of the peri-implant papillae. In Class 1, IHB is 4–5 mm (measured from the apical extent of future contact point of the restoration to the crest of

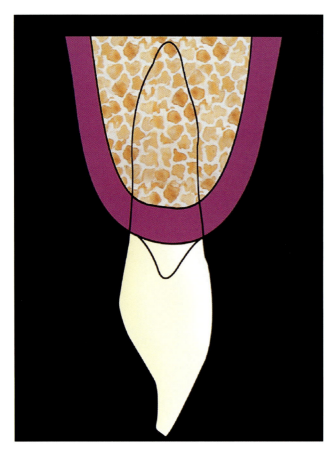

FIGURE 4.33c.   Class III Nordland classification.

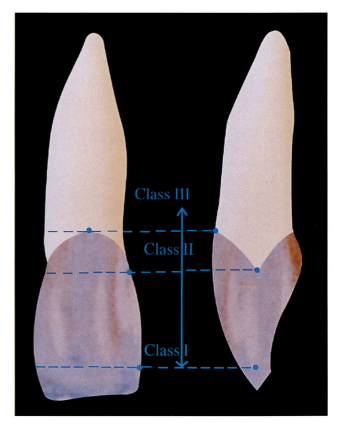

FIGURE 4.33d.   Nordland classification legend.

bone), suggesting an optimal prognosis; Class 2 shows an IHB of 6–7 mm with a guarded prognosis; and in Class 3 IHB is greater than 7 mm, indicating a poor prognosis (Fig. 4.35).

Basic Morphology of the Interproximal Papillae

The clinical configuration of the interdental papilla basically depends on the volume of the underlying osseous support and the morphology of the proximal surfaces of the adjacent teeth. The osseous structure of the interdental papilla is composed of two crests or peaks from the labial and lingual sides. The labial crest is slightly higher than the lingual one, with an intervening distance of 2–6 mm. The two crests are connected by the so-called gingival col, which may be convex or concave in shape, or have a sawlike appearance.[165]

Histologically, the interdental papilla is composed of stratified squamous epithelium covering its crest,[157] with abundant bundles of collagenous fibers running through the lamina propria. The collagenous fibers, which run in a buccolingual direction through the lamina propria,[166–168] may have a significant role in keeping the marginal

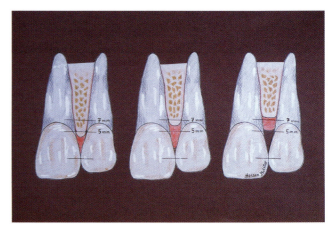

FIGURE 4.34.   Tarnow et al. classification to assess predictability of interdental papillae.

gingiva closely adherent to the neck of the tooth; thus these fibers are responsible for maintaining both the shape and the position of the papilla. The connective tissue contains lymphocytes and plasma cells.

Different terms have been coined to identify or distinguish between the interproximal papillae located at different sites. The papilla that exists between natural dentition is called *interdental papilla*, that located

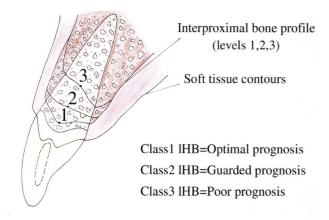

Interproximal bone profile
(levels 1,2,3)

Soft tissue contours

Class1 IHB=Optimal prognosis
Class2 IHB=Guarded prognosis
Class3 IHB=Poor prognosis

FIGURE 4.35. Salama et al. classification of the interproximal height of bone.

between an implant and a natural tooth is *peri-implant papilla*, and if papilla exists between two adjacent implants, it is called *interimplant papilla*. When *papilla* is used in a generalized term (unspecified), it can be called *interproximal papilla*.

The soft tissue histological characteristics of interimplant papillae and interdental papillae are similar, except that interimplant papillae have a connective tissue fiber orientation,[18] have a high percentage of collagen fibers with fewer fibroblasts, and attain a less adequate blood supply because of the absence of the periodontal ligament.[169] This makes the interimplant papillae more like scar tissue, which may complicate any attempts for surgical repair or reconstruction. When the interimplant papilla is missing or does not totally fill the embrasure space, the condition looks like and is called a *black triangle*.

Peri-implant papillae are more clinically achievable than the interimplant papillae because the CEJ at the proximal surface of the adjacent natural tooth follows a reverse scalloping toward the incisal edge; this keeps the interproximal bone at the same height by means of Sharpey's fibers,[170] which is not the same as the situation for adjacent multiple implants.

Soft Tissue Procedures for Reconstruction of the Interimplant Papillae

The interimplant papillae are characterized by diminished blood supply, because of the histological nature of the peri-implant soft tissue and because of its marginal location. This explains the poor prognosis of any surgical reconstruction attempt. Several surgical procedures have been introduced in an attempt to solve the problem; among these soft tissue surgical procedures are coronally positioned flaps in combination with connective tissue

grafts,[171] coronally positioned palatal sliding flaps,[172] and Beagle's technique.[173]

Beagle's technique entails a palatal pedicle flap that is folded and tied on itself on the facial side in order to increase the height of the interimplant papilla. Regrettably, this method did not attain a high success rate because of the compromised blood supply of the small-sized pedicle (Fig. 4.36).

Alternatively, Han and Takei[171] described a technique that makes use of a pedicle graft with a semilunar incision and total coronal displacement of the gingival unit. Others have disclosed several methods for minimizing gingival recession around dental implants to improve the interimplant papilla contours. [51]

Azzi et al.[174] employed a connective tissue graft to be placed on the defective area then tucked under buccal and palatal flaps, thus providing the graft with an adequate blood supply (Fig. 4.37a–e). The method requires

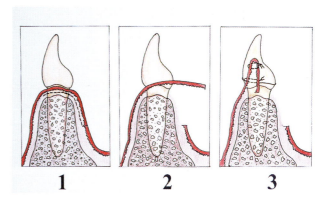

1 2 3

FIGURE 4.36. Beagle's technique.

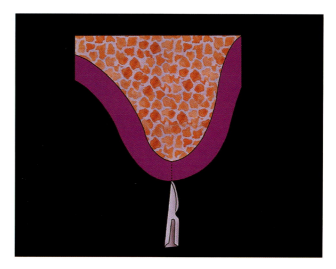

FIGURE 4.37a. Illustration showing Azzi et al. technique for regenerating the interdental papilla with a connective tissue graft.

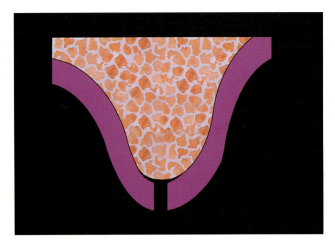

FIGURE 4.37b. Illustration showing the crestal incision.

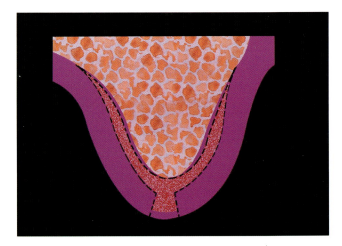

FIGURE 4.37e. The graft secured in place.

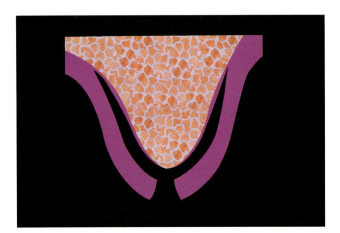

FIGURE 4.37c. Illustration showing the labial and lingual partial thickness flaps reflected.

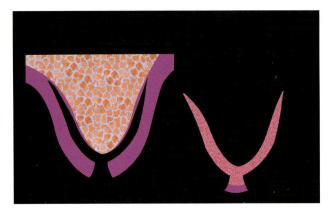

FIGURE 4.37d. Illustration showing the preparation of the composite connective tissue graft.

two buccal and lingual marginal partial thickness incisions at the compromised site. A wedge-shaped graft is harvested from the tuberosity. It is then shaped and

trimmed to obtain two connective tissue extensions with an epithelial crest on the center. When both flaps cover the connective tissue ends of the graft, the epithelial crest stays exposed to increase the height of the interimplant papilla.

Osseous Regenerative Methods for Interimplant Papillae

Based on Holmes findings,[157] the therapeutic techniques utilizing only soft tissue intervention to regenerate interimplant papillae did not attain predictable clinical results. It makes more sense to first regenerate the underlying osseous support. Hence, attention is turned towards regenerating the osseous structure of the interimplant papillae to regain the overall lost tissue height medially between implants.[155] This conclusion is confirmed by Salama et al.: "successful and predictable aesthetic results can be accomplished only when underlying labial and interproximal osseous support has been therapeutically provided."[164]

In an attempt to regenerate the osseous support of a deficient interimplant papilla, an interimplant papilla regenerative template has been introduced recently. Although the template is still in its preliminary experimental stages, it showed an acceptable clinical success.

Interimplant Papilla Regenerative Template

The interimplant papilla regenerative template[155] (Fig. 4.38) is a carrier fabricated from pure titanium. It acts as a housing that supports the bone-grafting material on the alveolar ridge, and it is placed between two implants to

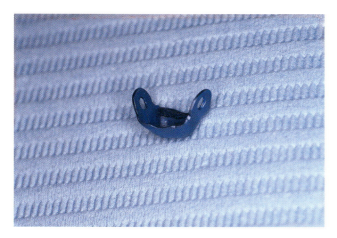

FIGURE 4.38. Interimplant papilla regenerative template.

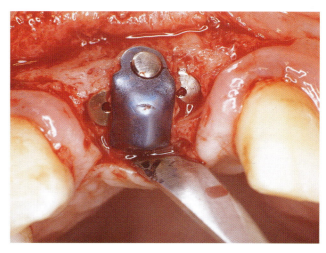

FIGURE 4.39a. The template carrying the bone-grafting material and secured in place with two fixation screws.

regenerate an osseous foundation for the interimplant papilla.

The template is to be placed at the time of implant insertion, therefore eliminating the need for any additional surgical procedure. Other advantages of the template are that it carries and protects the bone graft material and also separates the bone-grafting mix from the undesired fibroblast and epithelial cells, which favors graft predictability.

The use of the template requires a space of not less than 3 mm between two adjacent implants. After the implants are inserted, the interimplant bone is decorticated, to provide sufficient blood supply to the graft. [The grafting mix that is commonly used with the template is 50% autogenous bone chips harvested from the drilling procedure and 50% mineralized freeze-dried bone (Pacific Coast Tissue Bank, California, U.S.A.). Recently, however, the author has found that use of 100% autogenous chips can provide a more predictable clinical outcome. The template is then placed on the ridge with its two perforated ends facing the alveolar ridge. Two GBR fixation pins (IMTEC Corp., Ardmore, Oklahoma, U.S.A.) are fitted into the perforated ends of the template to stabilize the template and secure it in place. Soft tissue closure can be performed according to the previously mentioned protocol for soft tissue closure in critical conditions in this chapter (Fig. 4.39a–d).

At the time of the second-stage surgery, the template is removed, revealing the regenerated bone, and the flap is then sutured and left to heal. After soft tissue healing is complete, the provisional prosthesis is used to develop the emergence profile, as mentioned earlier. Use of smooth thin margins on the provisional prosthesis is mandatory in order to not exert pressure on the newly formed bone.

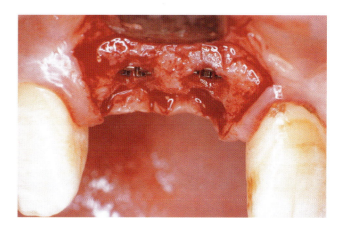

FIGURE 4.39b. The bone regenerated between the two implants after template removal in second-stage surgery.

The long-term prognosis of this method is still under investigation, as postoperative bone remodeling will be an important factor to be considered. This method requires further assessment and maybe a new generation of bone-grafting materials will help ensure more predicable results.

Prosthetic Solutions for Papillary Creation

Soft-tissue-colored acrylic stents were utilized long ago to solve many aesthetic problems associated with anterior fixed restorations on natural teeth; they might be used now to improve aesthetic and phonetic problems associated with losing interimplant papillae. Papillary illusions are yet another method used to modify the

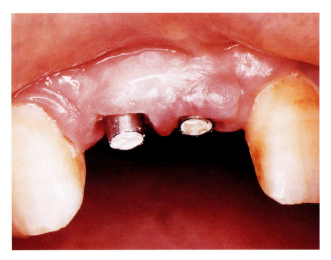

FIGURE 4.39c. The interimplant papilla is formed between the two implants.

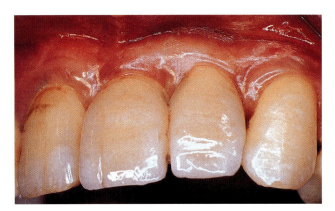

FIGURE 4.39d. Postoperative view showing the case finally restored.

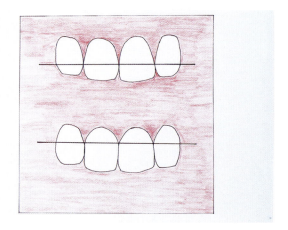

FIGURE 4.40. Papillary illusion.

final prosthesis by moving the contact area in an apical direction, thus making the gingival embrasures smaller in size and giving the impression that the interimplant papilla fills most of the gingival embrasure space. Prosthetic papillary illusion can be used in small and moderate losses of interimplant papilla. This method gives an acceptable clinical result without the need to perform any invasive surgical procedure (Fig. 4.40).

An alternative method, which requires a highly experienced dental technician, is the use of pink porcelain[175] to mimic the natural appearance of the papilla. With this method oral hygiene might be compromised, and the porcelain color usually does not match the color of the adjacent natural tissues.

A removable provisional prosthesis can influence the underlying gingival tissues at the pontic areas to create a papilla-like shape; this can be achieved by adding acrylic resin to the fitting surface of the pontic in order to press and conform the alveolar mucosa, forming a papilla between the two pontics. (Fig. 4.41a,b).

Noninvasive Methods for Papillary Reconstruction

Interestingly, Jemt[176] observed that the peri-implant papillae can regenerate without any clinical manipulation of the soft tissue to some extent one to three years after completing the implant therapy. He reasoned that plaque accumulation in the proximal areas causes gingival inflammation and hyperplasia, which sequentially leads to overgrowth of the papilla to fill the interproximal space. Creeping of interdental papilla on the tooth surface[171] as well as onto porcelain crowns[177,178] has been reported in the literature. Scaling and root planing also may induce proliferation of the gingival tissues (referred to as inflammatory hyperplasia).[179] This can lead to regeneration of the interdental papilla after nine months time. However, creeping of the interdental papilla around the root surface is not clinically predictable in many clinical conditions. Forced eruption[180,181] is another noninvasive method for regenerating interdental or peri-implant papillae. Development of the interdental papillae can be achieved by the application of a continuous light force; after a few months, coronal migration of the attachment apparatus occurs, as explained earlier in Chapter 2.

Future Methods for Papillary Reconstruction

Recently the soft tissue ballooning concept has been investigated as a technique for developing a subgingival tissue space that can be filled later with any commercially available silicon material or bone cement. Also, titanium papilla inserts were inserted subgingivally to regain the shape of the interimplant papilla.[155] Unfortunately, the delicate nature of the oral mucosa did not allow any success for these trials.

The current thought is to use mini osteodistraction devices to increase bone height in the future interimplant

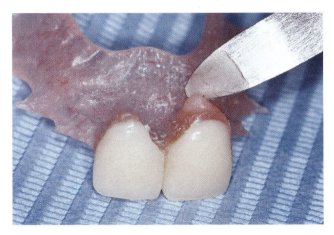

FIGURE 4.41a. Prosthetic solution to enhance the interdental papilla by adding a resin material to the fitting surface of the removable partial denture, in order to press and reshape the pontic area.

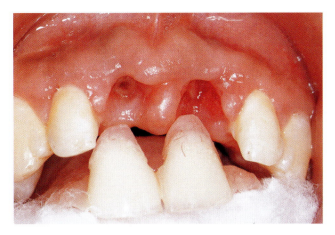

FIGURE 4.41b. The postconfiguration effect of the alveolar ridge pontic development.

papilla areas, or to distract all of the bone segment that will receive the implants to a higher level than the CEJ of the adjacent teeth. The distracted bone at the place of the future implants is reduced to its optimal height, while the bone sites for the future interimplant papillae are left as is, thus maintaining the required height of the interimplant papillae.[183] This method is still under investigation because the construction of mini osteodistractors will be expensive and the treatment time will be doubled, which is considered a handicapping factor.

CONCLUSION

Developing and regenerating the interimplant papillae is a challenging and difficult clinical task. Further research efforts are required to test and improve the current techniques. Most of the published data are case reports that lack long-term evaluations and predictable clinical results.[182] Careful treatment planning, optimal implant positioning, proper use of the provisional prostheses, and development of appropriate surgical skills are all factors that should be considered during dental implant therapy in the aesthetic zone.

REFERENCES

1. El Askary AS. The use of connective tissue grafts to enhance esthetics. J Prosthet Dent 2002 (87):129–132.
2. Croll BM. Emergence profiles in natural tooth contour. Part I: Photographic observations. J Prosthet Dent 1989(62): 374–379.
3. Alberktsson T and Hansson HA. An ultrastructural characterisation of the interface between bone and sput-tered titanium or stainless steel surfaces. Biomaterials 1986(7): 201–205.
4. Buser D, Schenk RK, Steinemann S, Fiorellini JP, Fox CH, and Stich H. Influence of surface characteristics on bone integration of titanium implants. A histomorphometric study in miniature pigs. J Biomed Mater Res 1991(25): 889–902.
5. Sennerby L, Thomsen P, and Ericson LE. Early bone tissue response to titanium implants inserted in rabbit cortical bone. I. Light microscopic observations. J Mat Sci Mat Med 1993(4): 240–250.
6. Strid KG. Radiographic procedures. In Brånemark P-I, Zarb KG, and Albrektsson T, eds. Tissue Integrated Prostheses. Osseointegration in Clinical Dentistry. Chicago: Quintessence, 1985.
7. Seibert J. Reconstruction of the partially edentulous ridge: Gateway to improved prosthetics and superior aesthetics. Pract Periodont Aesthet Dent 1993(5): 47–55.
8. Garber DA. The edentulous ridge and fixed prosthodontics. Compend Contin Educ Dent 1981(2): 212.
9. Wennström JL. Mucogingival therapy. Ann Periodontol 1996(1): 671–701.
10. Chee WWL, Cho GC, and Donovan TE. Restoration of the anterior edentulous space. J Calif Dent Assoc 1997(25): 381–385.
11. Chee WWL and Donovan TE. Treatment planning and soft tissue management for optimal implant aesthetics. Ann Acad Med Singapore 1995(24): 113–117.
12. El Askary AS. Esthetic considerations in anterior single tooth replacement. Implant Dent 1999(8): 61–67.
13. Stauts B. The anterior single-tooth implant restoration. J Calif Dent Assoc 1991(20): 35–40.
14. Neale D and Chee WWL. Development of soft tissue emergence profile: A technique. J Prosthet Dent 1994(71): 364–368.
15. Berman GR, Rapley JW, Hallmoon WW, et al. The peri-implant sulcus. Int J Oral Maxilofac Implants 1993(8): 273–280.

16. Abrahamsson I, Berglundh T, Glantz PO, and Lindhe J. The mucosal attachment at different abutment: An experimental study in dogs. J Clin Periodontol 1998(25): 721–727.

17. Akagawa Y, Takata T, Matsumoto T, Nikai H, and Tsuru H. Correlation between clinical and histological evaluations of the peri-implant gingiva around single-crystal sapphire endosseous implant. J Oral Rehabil 1989(16): 581–587.

18. Berglundh T, Lindhe J, Ericsson I, Marinello CP, Liljenberg B, and Thomsen P. The soft tissue barrier at implants and teeth. Clin Oral Implant Res 1991(2): 81–90.

19. Egelberg J. The blood vessels of the dento-gingival junction. J Periodontal Res 1966(1): 163–179.

20. Potashnick SR. Soft tissue modeling for the esthetic single-tooth implant restoration. J Esthet Dent 1998(10): 121–131.

21. Palacci P. Optimal implant positioning and soft-tissue considerations. Oral Maxillofac Surg Clin North Am 1996(8): 445–452.

22. Allen EP, Gainza CS, Farthing GG, and Newbold DA. Improved technique for localized ridge augmentation. A report of 21 cases. J Periodontol 1985(56): 195–199.

23. Seibert JS and Salama H. Alveolar ridge preservation and reconstruction. Periodontol 2000 1996(6): 69–84.

24. Israelsson H and Plemons JM. Dental implants, regenerative techniques, and periodontal plastic surgery to restore maxillary anterior esthetics. Int J Oral Maxillofac Implants 1993(8): 555–561.

25. Liljenberg B, Gualini F, Berglundh T, Tonetti T, and Lindhe J. Some characteristics of the ridge mucosa before and after implant installation: A prospective study in humans. J Clin Periodontol 1996(23): 1008–1013.

26. Moy PK, Weinlaender M, and Kenney EB. Soft tissue modifications of surgical techniques for placement and uncovering of osseointegrated implants. Dent Clin North Am 1989(33): 665–681.

27. Carlsson GE, Thilander H, and Hedegard G. Histologic changes in the upper alveolar process after extractions with or without insertion of an immediate full denture. Acta Odontol Scand 1967(25): 1–31.

28. Lazara RJ. Managing the soft tissue margin: The key to implant aesthetics. Pract Periodont Aesthet Dent 1993(5): 81–87

29. Small PN and Tarnow DP. Gingival recession around implants: A 1-year longitudinal prospective study. Int J Oral Maxillofac Implants 2000(15): 527–532.

30. El Askary AS. Multifaceted aspects of esthetic implantology. Implant Dent 2000(10): 182–191.

31. Tarnow DP, Eskow RN, and Zamok J. Aesthetics and implant dentistry. Periodontol 2000 1996(11): 85–94.

32. Seibert JS. Reconstruction of deformed, partially edentulous ridge, using full thickness onlay grafts. Part I. Technique and wound healing. Compendium1983(4): 437–453.

33. Langer B and Langer L. The subepithelial connective tissue graft technique for root coverage. J Periodontol 1985(56): 715–720.

34. Hurzeler MB and Dietmar W. Peri-implant tissue management: Optimal timing for an aesthetic result. Pract Periodont Aesthet Dent 1996(8): 857–869.

35. Langer B. Spontaneous in situ gingival augmentation. Int J Periodont Rest Dent 1994(14): 525–535.

36. Pietrokovski J and Massler M. Alveolar ridge resorption following tooth extraction, J Prosthet Dent 1967(17): 21–27.

37. Lam RV. Contour changes of the alveolar process following extraction. J Prosthet Dent 1960(10): 25–32.

38. Atwood DA. Postextraction changes in the adult mandible as illustrated by microradiographs of mid-sagittal sections and serial cephalometric roentgenograms. J Prosthet Dent 1963(13): 810–842.

39. Roberts EW, Turley PK, Brezneak N, et al. Bone physiology and metabolism. J Calif Dent Assoc 1987(15): 54–61.

40. Garretto LP, Chen J, Parr JA, et al. Remodeling dynamics of bone supporting rigidly fixed titanium implants. A histomorphometric comparison in four species including human, Implant Dent 1995(4): 235–243.

41. Landsberg CJ. Socket seal surgery combined with immediate implant placement: A novel approach for single-tooth replacement. Int J Periodont RestDent 1997(17): 141–149.

42. Landsberg CJ and Bichacho N. A modified surgical/prosthetic approach for optimal single implant supported crown. Part I—The socket seal surgery. Pract Periodont Aesthet Dent 1994(6): 11–17.

43. Dahlin C, Lindhe A, Gottlow J, and Nyman S. Healing of bone defects by guided tissue regeneration. Plast Reconstr Surg 1988(8)1: 672.

44. Misch CE, Misch FD, and Misch CM. A modified socket seal surgery with composite graft approach. J Oral Implantol 1999(4): 244–250.

45. Dahlin C, Alberius P, and Linde A. Osteopromotion for cranioplasty. An experimental study in rats using a membrane technique. J Neurosurg 1991(74): 487.

46. Hammack BL and Enneking WF. Comparative vascularization of autogenous and homogenous bone transplants, J Bone Joint Surg 1960(42A): 811.

47. Male AJ, Gasser J, Fonseca RJ, et al. Comparison of only autogous and allogenic bone grafts to the maxilla in primates, J Oral Maxillofac Surg 1983(42): 487–499.

48. Howes R, Bowness JM, Grotendorst GR, Martin GR, and Reddi AH. Platelet derived growth factor enhances demineralized bone matrix and induces cartilage and bone formation. Calcif Tissue Int 1988(42): 34–38.

49. Becker W and Becker B. Flap designs for minimization of recession adjacent to maxillary anterior sites, a clinical study, Int J Oral Maxillofac Implants 1996(11): 46–54.

50. Palacci P. Peri-implant soft tissue management: Papilla regeneration technique. In Palacci P, Ericsson I, Engstrand P, et al., eds. Optimal Implant Positioning and Soft Tissue Management for the Brånemark System. Chicago: Quintessence, 1995, 59–70.

51. Israelson H and Plemons JM, Dental implant, regenerative techniques and periodontal plastic surgery to restore —Maxillary anterior esthetics. Int J Oral Maxillofac Implants 1993(8): 555–561.

52. Block MS and Kent JN, Endosseous Implants for Maxillofacial Reconstruction. Philadelphia: W. B. Saunders, 1995.

53. Brånemark P-I, Zarb GA, and Albrektsson T, eds. Tissue-integrated Prostheses: Osseointegration in Clinical Dentistry. Chicago: Quintessence, 1985.

54. Buser D, Weber HP, and Long NP. Tissue integration of nonsubmerged implants: One-year results of a prospective study with 100 ITI hollow-screw and hollow-cylinder implants. Clin Oral Impl Res 1990(1): 33–40.

55. Weber HP, Buser D, Donath K, et al. Comparison of healed tissues adjacent to submerged and non-submerged unloaded titanium dental implants. A histometric study in beagle dogs. Clin Oral Implant Res 1996(7): 11–19.

56. Brägger U, Häfeli U, Huber B, et al. Evaluation of postsurgical crestal bone levels adjacent to non-submerged dental implants. Clinl Oral Implant Res 1998(9): 218–224.

57. Brånemark P-I, Hansson BO, Adel R, et al. Osseointegrated implants in the treatment of the edentulous jaw. Experience from the 10-year period. Scand J Plastic Reconstr Surg 1977 11(Suppl. 16): 1–132.

58. Misch CE, Progressive bone loading. Pract Period Esthet Dent 1990(2): 27–30.

59. Brunski JB et al. The influence of functional use of endosseous dental implants on the tissue-implant interface. II. Clinical aspects. J Dent Res 1979(58): 1970–1980.

60. Boss JH, Shajrawi I, and Mendes DG. The nature of the bone-implant interface. Med Prog Technol 1994(20): 119–142.

61. Bahat O and Handelsman M. Periodontal reconstructive flaps—Classification and surgical considerations. Int J Periodontics Restorative Dent 1991(11): 481–487.

62. Dahlberg WH. Incisions and suturing. Some basic considerations about each in periodontal flap surgery. Dent Clin North Am 1969(13): 149.

63. Johnson RH, Basic flap management, Dent Clin North Am 1976(20): 3.

64. Corn H. Mucogingival surgery and associated problems. In Goldman HM and Cohen DW, eds. Periodontal Therapy, 5th ed. St Louis: Mosby, 1973, 638–751.

65. McKinney RV, Jr. Endosteal Dental Implants. In Shelton DW, ed. Basic Surgical Principles for Implantology. St. Louis: Mosby Yearbook, 1991, 75–87.

66. Knox R, Caudill R, and Meffert R, Histologic evaluation of dental endosseous implants placed in surgically created extraction defects. Int J Periodontics Restorative Dent 1991(11): 365–375.

67. Esposito M, Hirsch JM, Lekholm U, et al. Biological factors contributing to failures of osseointegrated oral implants. I. Success criteria and epidemiology. Eur J Oral Sci 1998(106): 527–551.

68. Scharf DR and Tarnow DP. The effect of crestal versus mucobuccal incisions on the success rate of implant osseointegration. Int J Oral Maxillofac Implants 1993(8): 187–190.

69. Cranin AN, Klein M, Sirakian A, et al. Comparison of incisions made for the placement of dental implants. J Dent Res 1991(70): 279.

70. Casino AJ, Harrison P, Tarnow DP, et al. The influence of type of in incision on the success rate of implant integration at stage II uncovering surgery. J Oral Maxillofac Surg 1997(55): 31–37.

71. Hunt BW. Effect of flap design on healing and osseointegration of dental implants. Int J Periodontics Restorative Dent 1996(16): 582–593.

72. Kirkland O. Surgical flap and semilunar technique in periodontal surgery. Dent Digest 1936(42): 125.

73. Evian CI, Corn H, and Rosenberg ES. Retained interdental procedures for maintaining anterior esthetics. Compend Contin Educ Dent 1985(1): 58–65.

74. Wilderman MN. Exposure of bone in periodontal surgery. Dent Clin North Am 1964(3): 23–36.

75. Pennel BM, King KO, Wilderman MN, and Barron JM. Repair of the alveolar process following osseous surgery. J Periodontol 1967(38): 426–431.

76. Bragger U, Pasquali L, and Kornman KS. Remodeling of interdental alveolar bone after periodontal flap procedures assessed by means of computer-assisted densitometric image analysis (CADIA). J Clin Periodontol 1988(15): 558–564.

77. Elden A and Mejchar B. Plastic surgery of the vestibulum in periodontal therapy. Int Dent J 1963(13): 593.

78. Hertel RC, Blijdorp PA, and Bakter DL. A preventive mucosal flap technique for use in implantology. Int J Oral Maxillofac Implants 1993(8): 452–458.

79. Wilson TG, Schenk R, Buser D, and Cochran D. Implants placed in immediate extraction sites. A report of histometric analyses of human biopsies. Int J Oral Maxillofac Implants 1998(13): 333–341.

80. Werbitt MJ and Goldberg PV. The immediate implant: Bone preservation and bone regeneration. Int J Periodontics Restorative Dent 1992(12): 206–217.

81. Tehemar S. Assessment of heat generation in immediate implant procedure. J Oral Maxillofac Surg 1998 56(Suppl. 4): 36.

82. Lundgren D, Rylander H, Andersson M, et al. Healing-in of root analogue titanium implants placed into extraction sockets. An experimental study in the beagle dog. Clin Oral Implant Res 1992(3): 136–143.

83. Schabes GA, Sacks HG, and Kaufman PS. Osseointegrated fixture placement with simultaneous tooth extraction. Pract Periodont Aesthet Dent 1992(4): 37–42.

84. Lazarra RJ. Immediate implant placement into extraction sites: Surgical and restorative advantages. Int J Periodontics Restorative Dent 1989(9): 332–342.

85. Block MS and Kent IS. Placement of endosseous implants into tooth extraction sites. Int J Oral Maxillofac Surg 1991(49): 1269–1276.

86. Arlin ML. Immediate placement of osseointegrated dental implants into extraction sockets. Advantages and case reports. Oral Health 1992(82): 19–26.

87. Anneroth G, Hedström KG, Kjellman O, et al. Endosseous titanium implants in extraction sockets. An experimental study in monkeys. Int J Oral Surg 1985(14): 50–54.

88. Becker W and Becker BE. Guided tissue regeneration for implants placed into extraction socket and for implant dehiscences: Surgical techniques and case reports. Int J Periodontics Restorative Dent 1990(10): 376–391.

89. Gelb DA. Immediate implant surgery: Three-year retrospective evaluation of 50 consecutive cases. Int J Oral Maxillofac Implants 1993(8): 388–399.

90. Rosenquist B and Grenthe B, Immediate placement of implants into extraction sockets: Implant survival. Int J Oral Maxillofac Implants 1996(11): 205–209.

91. Gotfredsen K, Nimb L, Buser D, and Hjorting-Hansen E. Evaluation of guided bone regeneration around implants placed into fresh extraction sockets: An experimental study in dogs. J Oral Maxillofac Surg 1993(51): 879–884.

92. Gher ME, Quintero G, Assad D, et al. Bone grafting and guided bone regeneration for immediate implants in humans. J Periodontol 1994(65): 881–891.

93. Becker BE, Becker W, Ricci A, and Geurs N. A prospective clinical trial of endosseous screw-shaped implants placed at the time of tooth extraction without augmentation, J Periodontol 1998(69): 920–926.

94. Artzi Z and Nemcovsky C. Bone regeneration in extraction sites. Part 1: The simultaneous approach, Implant Dent 1997(6): 175–181.

95. Gher ME, Quintero G, Sandifer JB, et al. Combined dental implant and guided tissue regeneration therapy in humans. Int J Periodontics Restorative Dent 1994(14): 332–347.

96. Edel A. The use of a connective tissue graft for closure over immediate implants covered with an occlusive membrane. Clin Oral Implant Res 1995(6): 60–65.

97. Evian CI and Cutler S. Autogenous gingival grafts as epithelial barriers for immediate implants: Case reports. J Periodontol 1994(65): 201–210.

98. Becker W, Dahlin C, Becker BE, et al. The use of e-PTFE barrier membranes for bone promotion around titanium implants placed into extraction sockets: A prospective multicenter study. Int J Oral Maxillofac Implants 1994(9): 31–40.

99. Lekholm U, Becker W, Dahlin C, et al. The role of early versus late removal of GTAM membranes on bone formation at oral implants placed into immediate extraction sockets: An experimental study in dog. Clin Oral Implant Res 1993(4): 121–129.

100. Mellonig JT and Nevins M. Guided bone regeneration of bone defects associated with implants: An evidence-based outcome assessment. Int J Periodontics Restorative Dent 1995(15): 168–185.

101. Simion M, Baldoni M, Rossi P, and Zaffe D, A comparative study of the effectiveness of e-PTFE membranes with and without early exposure during the healing period. Int J Periodontics Restorative Dent 1994(14): 167–180.

102. Jovanovic SA, Spickerman H, and Richrer EJ, Bone regeneration around titanium dental implants in dehisced sites: A clinical study. Int J Oral Maxillofac Implants 1992(13): 29–45.

103. Hertel RC, Blijdorp PA, Kalk W, and Baker DL. Stage 2 surgical techniques in Endosseous Implantation. Int J Oral Maxillofac Implants 1994(9): 273–278.

104. Rosenquist B. A comparison of various methods of soft tissue management following the immediate placement of implants into extraction sockets. Int J Oral Maxillofac Implants 1997(12): 43–51.

105. Nemkovesky CE, Artzi A, and Moses O. Rotated palatal flap in immediate implant procedures. Clin Oral Implant Res 2000(11): 83–90.

106. Novaes AB, Jr and Novaes AB. Soft tissue management for primary closure in guided bone regeneration: Surgical technique and case report. Int J Oral Maxillofac Implants 1997(12): 84–87.

107. Von Rehrman A. Eine Methode zur Schliessung von Keiferhohlen Perforationen. Dtsch Zahnaerzth Wochenschr 1936(39): 1137.

108. Kay LW. The dental implications of the maxillary antrum. J Ir Dent Assoc 1970(16): 10–19.

109. Rosenquist B. Nouvelle technique chirurgicale d'implantation immediate a vocation esthetique. Implant 1996(2): 105–110.

110. Rosenquist BO and Ahmad M. The immediate replacement of teeth by dental implants using homologous bone membranes to seal the sockets: Clinical and radiographic findings. Clin Oral Implant Res 2000(11): 572–582.

111. al-Ansari BH and Morris RR. Placement of dental implants without flap surgery: A clinical report. Int J Oral Maxillofac Implants 1998(13): 861–865.

112. Landsberg CJ and Bichacho N. Implant placement without flaps: A single-stage surgical protocol—Part I. Pract Periodont Aesthet Dent 1998(10): 1033–1039.

113. Kan JK and Rungcharassaeng K. Immediate placement and provisionalization of maxillary anterior single implants: A surgical and prosthodontic rationale. Pract Periodont Aesthet Dent 2000(12): 817–824.

114. Becker W, Ochsenbein C, Tibbetts L, and Becker BE. Alveolar bone anatomic profiles as measured from dry skulls. Clinical ramifications. J Clin Periodontol 1997(24): 727–731.

115. Gottlow J, Nyman D, Lindhe J, Karring T, and Wennström J. New attachment formation in the human periodontium by guided tissue regeneration. Case reports. J Clin Periodontol 1986(13): 604–616.

116. Becker W, Becker B, Berg L, Prichard J, Caffesse R, and Rosenberg E. New attachment after treatment with root isolation procedures: Report for treated Class III and Class II furcation and vertical osseous defects. Int J Periodontics Restorative Dent 1988(8): 8–23.

117. Minabe M. Critical review of the biologic rational for guided tissue regeneration. J Periodontol 1991(62): 171–179.

118. Cochran DL, Hermann JS, Schenk RK, et al. Biologic width around titanium implants. A histometric analysis of the implant-gingival junction around unloaded and loaded nonsubmerged implants in the canine mandible. J Periodontol 1997(68): 186–198.

119. Bengazi F, Wennstrom JL, and Lekholm U. Recession of the soft tissue margin at oral implants. Clin Oral Implant Res 1996(7): 303–310.

120. Grunder U. Stability of the mucosal topography around single-tooth implants and adjacent teeth: One-year results. Int Periodontics Restorative Dent 2000(20): 11–17.

121. Schwarrz-Arad D and Chaushu G. Placement of implants into fresh extraction sites: 4 to 7 years retrospective evaluation of 95 immediate implants. J Periodontol 1997(68): 1110–1116.

122. Becker W, Becker BB, Polizzi G, and Bergstrom C. Autogenous bone grafting defects adjacent to implants placed into immediate extraction sockets in patients: A prospective study. Int J Oral Maxillofac Implants 1994(9): 389–396.

123. Landsberg CJ and Bichacho N. Implant placement without flaps: A single-stage protocol—Part 2. Utilizing a two-stage surgical protocol. Pract Periodont Asthet Dent 1999(11): 169–176.

124. Schwartz DA and Chaushu G. Immediate implant placement: A procedure without incisions. J Periodontol 1998(69): 743–750.

125. Auty C and Siddiqui A. Punch technique for preservation of interdental papillae at nonsubmerged implant placement. Implant Dent 1999(8): 160–166.

126. Esposito M, Hirsch JM, Lekholm U, et al. Biological factors contributing to failures of osseointegrated implants. II. Etiopathogenesis. Eur J Oral Sci 1998(106): 721–764.

127. Fugazzotto P. Maintenance of soft tissue closure following guided bone regeneration; technical considerations and report of 723 Cases. J Periodontol 1999(70): 1085–1097.

128. Langer B and Langer L. The overlapped flap: A surgical modification for implant fixture installation. Int J Periodontics Restorative Dent 1990(10): 209–216.

129. Fugazzotto PA, DePaoli S, and Benefenati SP. Flap design considerations in the placement of single maxillary anterior implants: Clinical report. Implant Dent 1993(2): 93–96.

130. Sclar A. Cosmetic soft-tissue enhancement for dental implants. Alpha Omegan 2000(93): 38–46.

131. Frisch J, Jones RA, and Bhastar SN. Conservation of maxillary anterior esthetics: A modified surgical approach. J Periodontol 1967(38): 11–17.

132. Takei HH, Yamada H, and Han TJ. Maxillary anterior esthetics. Preservation of the interdental papilla. Dent Clin North Am 1989(33): 263–273.

133. Takei HH, Han TJ, Carranza FA, Jr., Kenney EB, and Lekovic V. Flap technique for periodontal bone implants. Papilla preservation technique. J Periodontol 1985(56): 204–210.

134. Cortellini P, Pini Prato G, and Tonetti MS. The modified papilla preservation technique. A new surgical approach for interproximal regenerative procedures. J Periodontol 1995(66): 261–262.

135. Abrams L. Augmentation of the deformed residual edentulous ridge for fixed prosthesis. Compend Cont Educ Dept 1980(1): 205–213.

136. Seibert JS. Surgical preparation for fixed and removable prosthesis. In Genco RJ, Goldman HM, and Cohen DW, eds. Contemporary Periodontics. St. Louis: Mosby, 1990, 637–652.

137. Langer B and Calagna L. The subepithelial connective tissue graft. A new approach to the enhancement of anterior cosmetics. Int J Periodontics Restorative Dent 1982(2): 22–33.

138. Scharf DR and Tarnow DP. Modified roll technique for localized alveolar ridge augmentation. Int J Periodontics Restorative Dent 1992(12): 415–425.

139. El Askary AS. The use of connective tissue grafts to enhance esthetics. J Prosthet Dent 2001, in press.

140. Miller PD. Regenerative and reconstructive periodontal plastic surgery. Dent Clin North Am 1988(32): 287–306.

141. Seibert JS. Reconstruction of deformed, partially edentulous ridge, using full thickness onlay grafts. Part II. Prosthetic/periodontal interrelationships. Compend Cont Educ Dent 1983(4): 549–562.

142. Pennel BM, Tabor JC, King KO, Towner JD, Fritz BD, and Higgason JD. Free masticatory mucosa graft. J Periodontol 1969(40): 162–166.

143. Dordick B, Coslet JG, and Seibert JS. Clinical evaluation of free autogenous grafts placed on alveolar bone. Part I. Clinical predictability. J Periodontol 1976(47): 559–567.

144. Cohen ES. Atlas of Cosmetic and Reconstructive Periodontal Surgery, 2nd ed. Baltimore, MD: Lea & Febiger, 1994, 84–98.

145. Haeri A and Serio FG. Mucoginigval surgical procedures: A review of the literature. Quintessence Int 1999(30): 475–483.

146. Smukler H and Chaibi M. Ridge augmentation in preparation for conventional and implant supported restorations. Compendium 1994 18(Suppl.): 706–710.

147. Nabers J. Free gingival grafts. Periodontics 1966(4): 243–245.

148. James WC and Mc Fall WT. Placement of free gingival grafts on denuded alveolar bone. Part I: Clinical evaluations. J Periodontol 1978(49): 283.

149. Tarnow DP and Eskow RN, Preservation of implant esthetics: Soft and restorative considerations. J Esthet Dent 1995(8): 12–19.

150. Shulman J. Clinical evaluation of an acellular dermal allograft for increasing the zone of attached gingiva. Pract Periodont Aesthet Dent 1996(8): 203–208.

151. Nelson S. The subpedicle connective tissue graft. A bilaminar reconstructive procedure for the coverage of denuded root surfaces. J Periodontol 1987(58): 95–102.

152. Silverstein LH and Lefkove MD. The use of the subepithelial connective tissue graft to enhance both the aesthetics and periodontal contours surrounding dental implants. J Oral Implantol 1994(2): 135–138.

153. Allen EP. Pedicle flaps, gingival grafts, and connective tissue grafts in aesthetic treatment of gingival recession. Pract Periodont Aesthet Dent 1993(5): 29–38.

154. Bichacho N and Landsberg CJ. Single implant restoration: Prosthetically induced soft tissue topography. Pract Periodont Aesthet Dent 1997(9): 745–752.

155. El Askary AS. Inter-implant papilla reconstruction by means of a titanium guide. Implant Dent 2000(9): 85–89.

156. Engquist B, Nilson H, and Astrand P. Single tooth replacement by osseointegrated Brånemark implants. A retrospective study of 82 implants. Clin Oral Implant Res 1995(6): 238–245.

157. Holmes CH. Morphology of the interdental papillae. J Periodontol 1965(36): 455–460.

158. Tinti C, Vincenzi G, Cortellini P, Pinti Prato GP, and Clauser C. Guided tissue regeneration in the treatment of human facial recession. A 12-case report. J Periodontol 1987(58): 95–102.

159. Salama H, Salama M, Garber D, and Adar P. Developing optimal peri-implant papillae within the esthetic zone: Guided soft tissue augmentation. J Esthet Dent 1995(7): 125–129.

160. Miller PD, Jr. Root coverage using a free soft tissue autograft following citric acid application. Part I. Technique. Int J Periodontics Restorative Dent 1982(2): 65–70.

161. Harvey PM, Management of advanced periodontitis. Part I. Preliminary report of method of surgical reconstruction. N Z Dent J 1965(61): 180–187.

162. Nordland WP and Tarnow DP. A classification system for loss of papillary height. J Periodontol 1998(69): 1124–1126.

163. Tarnow DP, Magner AW, and Fletcher P. The effect of the distance from the contact point to the crest of the bone on the presence or absence of the interproximal dental papilla. J Periodontol 1992(63): 995–996.

164. Salama H, Salama MA, Garber D, and Adar P. The interproximal height of bone: A guidepost to predictable aesthetic strategies and soft tissues contours in anterior tooth replacement. Pract Periodont Aesthet Dent 1998(10): 1131–1141.

165. Cohen B. Morphological factors in the pathogenesis of periodontal diseases. Br Dent J 1959(107): 31–39.

166. Stahl S. Morphology and healing pattern of human interdental gingivae. J Am Dent Assoc 1963(67): 48.

167. Melcher A. The Interpapillary ligament. Dent Practitioner Dent Rec 1962(12): 461.

168. Arnim A and Hagerman D. The connective tissue fibers of the marginal gingiva. J Am Dent Assoc 1953(47): 271.

169. Berglundh T, Lindhe J, Jonsson K, and Ericsson I. The topography of the vascular system in the periodontal and peri-implant tissue in the dog. J Clin Periodontol 1994(21): 189–193.

170. Misch EC. Single tooth implant. In Misch CE, ed. Contemporary Implant Dentistry. St. Louis: Mosby, 1999, 397–428.

171. Han TJ and Takei HH. Progress in gingival papilla reconstruction. Periodontol 2000 1996(11): 65–68.

172. Tinti C and Parma-Benfenati S. Coronally positioned palatal sliding flap. Int J Periodontics Restorative Dent 1995(15): 298–310.

173. Beagle JR. Surgical reconstruction of the interdental papilla: Case report. Int J Periodontics Restorative Dent 1992(12): 145–151.

174. Azzi R, Etienne D, and Carranza F, Surgical reconstruction of the interdental papilla. Int J Periodontics Restorative Dent 1998(18): 467–473.

175. Cronin RJ and Wardle WL. Loss of anterior interdental tissue: Periodontal and prosthodontic solutions. J Prosthet Dent 1983(50): 505–506.

176. Jemt T. Regeneration of gingival papillae after single-implant treatment. Int J Periodontics Restorative Dent 1997(17): 327–333.

177. Matter J and Cimasoni G. Creeping attachment after free gingival grafts. J Periodontol 1976(47): 574–579.

178. Bell LA, Valluzzo TA, Garnick JJ, and Pennel BM. The presence of creeping attachment in human gingivae. J Periodontol 1978(49): 513–517.

179. Shapiro A. Regeneration of interdental papilla using periodic curettage. Int J Periodontics Restorative Dent 1985(5): 27–33.

180. Ingber JS. Forced eruption: Part I. A method of treating one and two wall infrabony osseous defects—Rationale and case report. J Periodontol 1974(45): 199–206.

181. Ingber JS. Forced eruption: Part II. A method of treating nonrestorable teeth—Periodontal and restorative considerations. J Periodontol 1976(47): 203–216.

182. Blatz MB, Hurzeler MB, and Strub JR. Reconstruction of the lost interproximal papilla—Presentation of surgical and nonsurgical approaches. Int J Periodontics Restorative Dent 1999(19): 395–406.

183. Moy P. Personal communications. Barcelona, Spain, 2002.

5
Aesthetic Bone Grafting

Luc Huys
Abd El Salam El Askary

INTRODUCTION

Healthy osseous structure of the alveolar ridge maintains the aesthetic soft tissue appearance around natural dentition and provides a framework for peri-implant soft tissue contours. Lack of alveolar bone, especially in the maxilla due to postextraction bone resorption, can result in functional and aesthetic problems that necessitate the use of augmenting procedures to reestablish the missing original dimensions. The advent of novel osseous regenerative techniques has significantly increased the functional and aesthetic potential of dental implants by restoring alveolar ridge defects to their original dimensions, which allows for optimal implant placement[1,2] and, in turn, increases the credibility of dental implant therapy as a unique treatment alternative.

Osseous reconstruction of the alveolar ridge can be classified according to its goal, either functional or aesthetic. Jovanovic[3] has divided the locations in the oral cavity into (1) aesthetically visible locations where adequate osseous structure (that supports the peri-implant soft tissue to develop a natural emergence profile) is important in obtaining aesthetic and functional results and (2) nonaesthetically visible locations where adequate osseous support is required to ensure long-term functional success.

The underlying osseous structure influences the shape and appearance of the investing soft tissues. Unfortunately, in the anterior maxilla the osseous structure of the alveolar bone undergoes a rapid process of postextrac-

tion resorption. It loses almost 25% of its volume during the first year and up to 40–60% in width within the first three years after tooth loss.[1,2] Therefore, many osseous reconstructive techniques have been introduced to help restore alveolar ridge defects. Recently, the term *aesthetic bone-grafting procedures* was introduced to define the aesthetic dimension of bone-grafting prodecures; it refers to the regeneration of the missing osseous structure to support the future aesthetic gingival contours while maintaining long-term implant success at the same time.[3,4] Therefore, restoring the lost volume of the underlying hard tissues either prior to or simultaneously with the implant placement can maintain and support not only an aesthetic implant-supported restoration but also the related facial structures.[5,6]

The variations in maxillary alveolar bone resorption patterns require different treatment approaches; the size and type of each particular osseous defect influence the selection of the most suitable grafting procedure. For example, minor alveolar ridge defects suggest the use of an allografting material in a nonstaged surgical approach, while moderate horizontal ridge defects require the use of more predictable grafting procedures such as autogenous grafts in a staged treatment approach.[3,7–9] In cases of combined severe horizontal and vertical alveolar ridge defects, the use of reconstructive devices will be mandatory to ensure more predictable regenerative results.[10,11]

The technological advancements in intraoral bone-grafting procedures are immense. One of the current developments in bone-grafting techniques involves using bone morphogenetic proteins (BMPs), such as BMP-2, on a collagen carrier[12] to enhance the predictability of the regenerated bone and to increase the bone density through a slow resorption and remodeling process. The BMP-2 helps increase local stem cell mitosis to recruit undifferentiated mesenchymal cells to the grafted site. These cells may be transformed to osteoblasts, by the

---

Dr. Luc W.S. Huys, is a professor at the Flemish Institute for Orthomolecular Sciences in Belgium. Dr. Huys is also the cofounder of the International Acacemy of Replacement Therapy.

appropriate morphogenetic cytokine, and start the bone matrix formation process.[13,14] This process is called the multiple type mitogen-morphogen mechanism for stimulating osseous healing. It may become the ideal bone-grafting procedure in the near future.[15]

Technical advancements have also taken place in the manufacture of the guided bone regenerative barriers[16,17]; these advancements have been mainly focused on the enhancement of the physical characteristics and biocompatibility of the barrier materials. Many types of barriers are available in the market and are made either resorbable (e.g., collagen membranes or membranes of polylactic acid alone, polylactic acid combined with polyglycolic acid, or polylactic acid in its polymer form) or nonresorbable (e.g., polytetrafluoroethylene or its expanded or reinforced forms). The resorbable biodegradable membranes require less tissue manipulation and seem to elicit less tissue reaction due to their biological nature.[18–21] The nondegradable membranes stay longer in the grafted site, thus providing a long-term regenerative effect, but require a second surgery for removal.[22–24] However, the litrature did not provide a definite answer on which of the two material types is more predictable.[25] Selection of suitable guided bone regenerative barriers should be based on a thorough understanding of the inherent benefits and limitations of the material in relation to the functional requirements of the specific clinical applications.[26]

Autogenous bone grafting in any reconstructive procedure is considered to be the gold standard of all bone-grafting procedures, because it provides proteins such as bone-enhancing substrates, minerals, and vital bone cells to the recipient site, which enhance the overall success of the grafting procedure, resulting in high success rates.[27–30] Sites used for harvesting autogenous bone for alveolar bone grafting can be either extraoral or intraoral. Extraoral harvesting sites include the posterior iliac crest of the hip and the calvaria,[31,32] but unfortunately, extraoral grafts showed a higher rate of morbidity than intraoral grafts and required complex surgery.[33] On the other hand, intraoral sites, such as the maxillary tuberosity, the ascending ramus, and particularly the symphysis of the mandible, offer better quality of cancellous and cortical bone and more predictable postoperative results.[34]

Recently, in 1996, distraction osteogenesis was introduced as a promising method for restoring a defecient alveolar ridge to its size.[35,37] The technique has been taken from orthopedic surgery, as used in the elongation of tubular bone in children, and now is predictably used in restoring severe atrophy of the alveolar ridge.[36,38] It eliminates the need for donor site surgery and reduces the risk of morbidity in comparison with the autogenous grafting procedures.[39]

Selection of the appropriate grafting technique or grafting material influences the success and predictability of the final treatment outcome. Defect size and type and the patient's general health condition are some factors that influence the decision making in bone-grafting procedures.

THE REPAIR PROCESS

Surgical intervention always produces a trauma that is repaired via a complex biological process that consists of three phases that will overlap one another in time: (1) the inflammatory (or exudative phase), (2) the proliferative phase, and the (3) repair phase.[40] The first phase starts with homeostasis, which is triggered by the interaction of vessel walls, platelets, and coagulation factors. The result of this interaction is a "coagulum" that becomes colonized by inflammatory cells within two to four hours, followed by fibroblasts within twenty-four to thirty-six hours. The three-dimensional fibrin net, which constitutes the framework of the coagulum, acts as a guide for cellular colonization.[40,41] During this phase, cellular necrosis (resulting from the surgical trauma) and homeostasis (resulting from the hemorrhage) produce and liberate numerous factors that trigger the migration of inflammatory cells into the defect, creating the necessary conditions for healing. Chemotactic factors that act on the leucocytes, present in the extravascular spaces, will influence the migration of inflammatory cells toward of the inflammatory stimulus.[40,41] Lysosomal enzymes provoke vasodilatation, which in turn provokes slowing of the blood flow that permits the leucocytes to migrate towards the vessel walls, adhere to them, and penetrate through them. Growth factors, produced by macrophages (derived from the transformation of monocytes) during their function of cellular debris removal induce the second phase.[40–42]

The proliferative phase is characterized by the reproduction of the fibroblasts as a result of the chemotactic attraction by the growth factors. It also has a role in synthesizing collagen. Platelets assist the macrophages to secrete factors that favor tissue repair. Platelets act indirectly by attracting macrophages and fibroblasts, and directly by stimulating replication of fibroblasts and collagen synthesis.[40–42]

The third phase, repair, is characterized by a marked increase in the synthesis of collagen with the complete formation of fibrous tissue as a substitute for the tissue damaged during the surgical procedure.[40–42]

In the presence of an implanted graft material the repair process undergoes a different tissue reaction that deviates from the normal process, especially in its intensity and duration.[42] An accumulation of extracellular fluid that contains proteins and inflammatory cells surrounds the implanted material. The proteins are absorbed at the surface of the implanted graft and undergo a variation of their configuration to an extent that they condition the functional response of the peri-implant cells.[42] The inflammatory cells can then modify the structure, the physical and chemical properties, of the surface of the graft material, usually causing a foreign body giant cell reaction, which activates the macrophages and leads to the production of cytokines that stimulate the production of collagen and bone tissue.[40–42]

A layer of fibrous connective tissue will surround graft material as it will any other device that remains for a certain time in the body. The surrounding fibrous tissue layer attains different thicknesses and shapes depending on its location, the mechanical stimuli, and the chemical characteristics of the graft interface.[40–42]

If the implanted graft material is biocompatible, the alterations in the repair process are limited, and the presence of fibrosis (which typically characterizes the final phase) is minimal. Biocompatibility can be defined as the capacity of a material to function in a specific application and provoke an appropriate reaction by the host.[42] Therefore, biocompatibility should involve the chemical and physical characteristics of the bone grafting material in order to avoid systemic or local toxicity and carcinogenic or genotoxic reactions.[40–42]

MECHANISMS OF BONE REGENERATION

Bone regeneration can be accomplished through three different mechanisms: osteogenesis, osteoinduction, and osteoconduction.[43–46] Osteogenesis is the formation and development of bone, even in the absence of local undifferentiated mesenchymal stem cells.[43] Osteogenic grafts can facilitate the different phases of bone regeneration, thus activating a faster osseous regeneration rate in most of the cases. An osteogenic graft is an organic material that is derived from, or composed of, living human tissue and is harvested from the individual in whom it will be used.[43] Osteoinduction is the transformation of undifferentiated mesenchymal stem cells into osteoblasts or chondroblasts through growth factors that exist only in living bone. Osteoinductive grafts enhance and facilitate normal bone regeneration, or even extend the regenerative process sometimes in places where it is not normally found.[43] Osteoconduction is the process that provides a bioinert scaffold, or physical matrix, suitable for the deposition of new bone.[43–46] Osteoconductive grafts (which are often inorganic) allow bone apposition from the surrounding bone or encourage differentiated mesenchymal cells to grow along the graft surface. They do not stimulate bone formation when placed in soft tissues.

All grafting materials have one or more of these three mechanisms of action. The mechanisms by which the grafts act are normally determined by their origin and composition.

TYPES OF BONE-GRAFTING MATERIALS

There are four forms of bone-grafting material: autogenous grafts, allografts, xenografts, and alloplasts.

Autogenous Grafts

Of all the bone-grafting materials, autogenous bone is still regarded as the "gold standard," because it is the only osteogenic grafting material.[43,46] Grafted autogenous bone heals through osteogenesis, osteoinduction, and osteoconduction, and those stages overlap during the healing process.[43] Autogenous bone grafts can be harvested from extraoral sites such as the iliac crest, the cranial bones, or the ribs; from intraoral sites such as the mandibular symphysis, the maxillary tuberosity, the ramus, and bone exostoses; and sometimes from the osteotomy drilling procedure. Its organic component, collagen, which provides the resilience, strength, and stability for the graft, whereas the inorganic component, hydroxyapatite, contributes to the rigidity of the graft. Grafted autogenous bone can be trabecular, cortical, or corticotrabecular. Trabecular grafts provide numerous osteogenic cells in their structure, while a cortical graft has fewer surviving osteogenic cells but provides the most bone morphogenetic protein (BMP), the essential agent for bone formation.[47] BMP differentiates host mesenchymal cells into osteoblasts.[47–49] In addition, BMP provides more resistance to the graft structure, which impedes soft tissue in-growth but also may prolong the time needed for blood vessels to infiltrate the graft.[47–49] Corticotrabecular grafts can be shaped and trimmed to fit the recipient bed, and the trabecular part is placed to face the recipient bed.

The healing process follows one of three paths: (1) the graft becomes viable, acquiring in time the characteristics of adjacent bone, (2) the graft resorbs partially or completely, resulting in instability, or (3) the graft becomes sequestrated and is treated by the host as a foreign body.[43,46]

Autogenous bone grafts are highly osteogenic and best fulfill, in theory, the requirements for bone regeneration. However, they possess some important practical shortcomings:

- Harvesting of the graft requires an additional surgery, which increase the patient postoperative inconvenience.
- Another osseous defect at the donor site is created, which presents an extra risk of infection and/or morbidity.

- Extensive graft resorption can be expected, especially with iliac grafts, but less with mandibular grafts (because they are from the same embryonic origin as the recipient site).
- Only limited amounts of graft material can be harvested from the intraoral donor sites.
- The possibility of apical root injury (in chin grafts) or sensory nerve damage exists.

These shortcomings have led to the development and use of other readily available grafts (allografts, xenografts, and alloplasts) that can be treatment alternatives used routinely and safely in the dental office (Fig. 5.1 a–g).

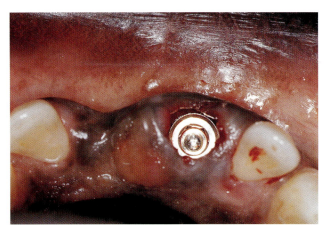

FIGURE 5.1a. Intraoperative view of a patient with an immediate implant (TSV Paragon, Centerpulse, Dental Division, Carlsbad, California) replacing the maxillary right central incisor; the place of the missing left central incisor shows an osseous defect that warrants grafting.

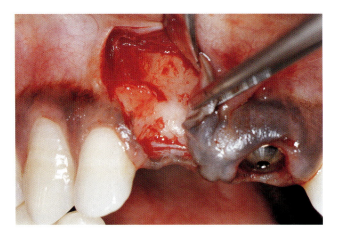

FIGURE 5.1b. A conservative mucoperiosteal flap is used to place an implant to restore the missing left central incisor and simultaneously graft the area. Note the conservation of the interimplant papilla and the peri-implant papilla in the flap design.

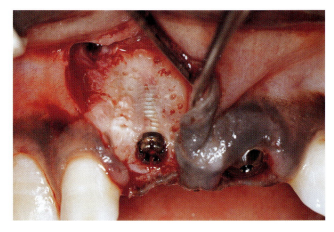

FIGURE 5.1c. An implant (Twist MP1, Centerpulse, Dental Division, Carlsbad, California) is placed within a dehiscent labial bone, with the cortical bone being decorticated.

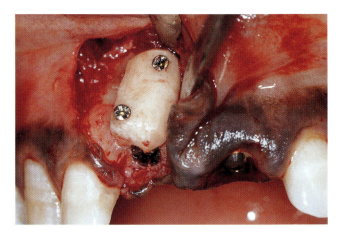

FIGURE 5.1d. A corticocancellous graft is harvested from the chin and fixed on top of the implant with two fixation screws. Note the place of the screws (lateral to the implant body).

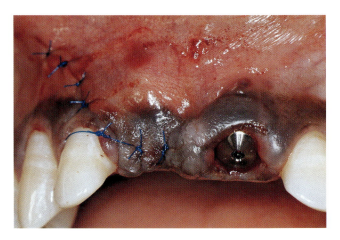

FIGURE 5.1e. Primary tension-free wound closure.

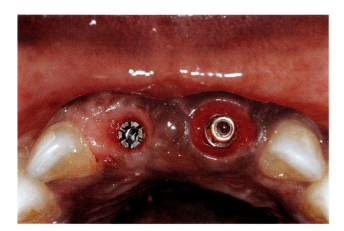

FIGURE 5.1f. Seven months postoperative view showing a remarkable improvement in the labial bone contour.

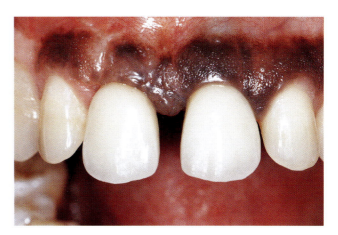

FIGURE 5.1g. The case finally restored.

Allografts

Allografts are obtained from other individuals of the same species, but from disparate genotypes.[43,45] Donors can be living related persons, living unrelated persons, or cadavers. The grafts are processed under completely sterile conditions and stored in bone banks. Transplanted bone allografts always induce a host immune response. To reduce this response, the nature of the bone graft is altered; three types of grafts are used: freeze-dried bone allografts (FDBAs), demineralized freeze-dried bone allografts (DFDBA), and irradiated cancellous bone allografts (ICBA). In a FDBA, the graft is dried at low temperature (lyophilized) without any liquid phase in the whole process. In a DFDBA the mineral phase of the FDBA is removed, exposing the collagen and the BMP. Without removal of this mineral phase, no bone induction process will be seen. Cortical bone chips are mostly preferred because of their low antigenic activity and the relatively large quantity of collagen. However, sterilization by gamma radiation kills most of the BMP present.[45] A DFDBA may regenerate bone by osteoinduction, by its effect on the host's undifferentiated mesenchymal cells while blood vessels penetrate the graft. DFDBAs may also regenerate bone by osteoconduction, by serving as a scaffold for the host bone while resorbing. However, Rummelhart et al. did not find any significant differences between the efficacy of FDBAs and DFDBAs in promoting bone repair of human periodontal defects six months postoperative.[50]

Irradiated cancellous bone has been used more recently. In its initial preparation, the bone was exposed to 6–8 million rads of radiation. Nowadays trabecular bone obtained from the spinal column can be treated only with 2.5 million rads.[46] Tatum reported that this material provided a response closest to autogenous bone.[46] The expense and morbidity involved with autogenous extraoral grafts made irradiated cancellous bone the most effective, readily available graft material that he has used.[46]

The advantages of allografts include ready availability, elimination of donor site surgery, reduced anesthesia and surgical time, and decreased blood loss.[43] Disadvantages consist primarily of the history of the obtained grafting material. The quality of the graft material depends mainly on the donor's health condition; for example, not having a history of infection, cancer, degenerative bone disease, hepatitis B or C, sexually transmitted disease, autoimmune deficiency, or other medical problems that might lead to cross infection.[43-45] Therefore, first priority must be given to thorough donor screening, which involves a traceable medical, demographic, and social history. Other disadvantages of allografts include the risk of rejection, high rate of infection, nonunion, risk of rapid resorption, and problems related to the considerable technical precision required to pack and hold the graft in place in bleeding sites (Figs. 5.2 and 5.3).[45,51]

To minimize the above-mentioned risks, Puros™ Allograft with Tutoplast® processing (Centerpulse, Dental division, Inc., Carlsbad, California, U.S.A.) recently has been introduced. The processing of the graft material consists of five stages (delipidization, osmotic contrast treatment, oxidation, solvent dehydration, and limited-dose of gamma irradiation), which are claimed to significantly reduce antigens and reactive agents.

In stage one, the graft is bathed in acetone and agitated with ultrasound. This removes fat (which interferes with healing), inactivates viruses, and prepares the graft so that the subsequent treatments penetrate the graft more effectively. In stage two, the osmotic contrast treatment, which is considered unique to the Tutoplast® processing, the graft receives alternating baths of distilled

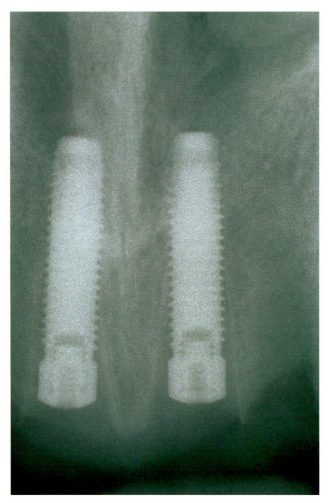

FIGURE 5.2. Placement of two immediate implants in fresh extracted sockets.

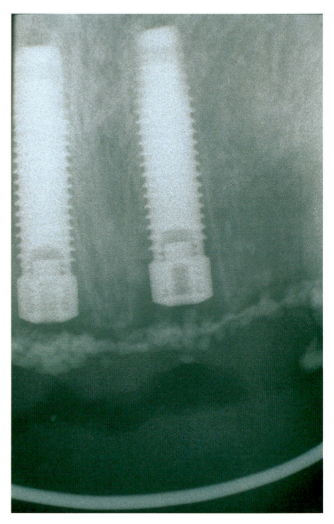

FIGURE 5.3. Radiographic view after application of a demineralized freeze-dried bone allograft; note that there is no grafting material around the neck of the implants or in the extraction sockets; the graft is held in place via a resorbable membrane.

water and saline. This might disrupt the cell wall integrity and exposes intracellular material. Bacteria are killed, undesirable cells are destroyed and removed (and as a result, so is most antigenicity), and the viral load is further reduced. During stage three, the graft is bathed in a hydrogen peroxide (H_2O_2) wash, destroying the remaining proteins, removing the residual antigenicity, inactivating any remaining viruses, and minimizing the potential for graft rejection. In stage four, the graft receives no less than seven acetone baths. This removes all the water, making the graft storable at room temperature, and preserves the dense collagen fibrous structure and its original strength. Finally, during the last stage, the graft receives a low-dose (17.8 kGy) gamma radiation, inactivating all remaining viruses and guaranteeing sterility following cutting and packaging.

Nevertheless, a rapidly increasing body of evidence questions the clinical relevance and the osteoinductive, osteoconductive, and regenerative potential of allograft materials after such bone preparations.[52-54]

Xenografts

Xenografts are obtained from a species other than the host species. The representative materials are natural hydroxyapatite and deorganified bovine bone. Natural hydroxyapatite is synthesized (by hydrothermal processing) from the calcium carbonate ($CaCO_3$) skeleton of coral.[44] It has the three-dimensional microstructure of natural bone with average pore sizes of 200 μ. It has approximately 60% void spaces and a calcium to phosphorus ratio of 10:6. The material is highly biocompatible and bonds readily to adjacent hard and soft tissues.

Thanks to its highly organized and permeable porous structure, with an interconnected three-dimensional architecture, the graft and the ingrown bone are remodeled in response to the same chemical and biomechanical forces that remodel normal bone. Its compressive strength increases following tissue ingrowth and is claimed to be sufficient to withstand masticatory forces exerted by dentures.[55,56] Reported disadvantages of this material are that the strength decreases exponentially with the increase in porosity, it is brittle and difficult to handle, the material migrates under stress during the healing period, and the material can only be used in non-infectious sites.[46]

Deorganified bovine bone is an inorganic bone of bovine origin. The graft is chemically treated to remove all organic components (calcium deficient carbonate-apatite) by heat processing. This process differs according to the material processed. That is, Osteograf/N® (CeraMed Dental, Lakewood, Colorado, U.S.A.) uses a high heat (1100°C) sintering process, resulting in fusion of bone crystallites, with decreased porosity and surface area. To enhance the cell-binding activity of this material, a new synthetic peptide analogous to a potent cell-binding domain in type I collagen, PepGen P-15™ (CeraMed Dental, Lakewood, Colorado, U.S.A.), is now promoted for use in combination with Osteograf®. The other chemical extraction process is done at low heat (300°C), and as a result, the exact trabecular architecture and porosity are maintained. When the graft is processed at low heat (Bio-Oss®; Geistlich AG, Wolhusen, Switzerland), it maintains the same compact apatite crystalline natural structure (Figs. 5.4 and 5.5). This similarity is important for remodeling (substitution of bone for bone as part of the natural growth process), which is needed for any graft to attain a degree of permanency.[57] Bio-Oss® is

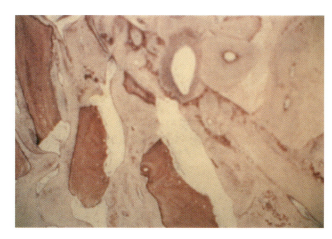

FIGURE 5.6. Figure demonstrating the integration of deorganified bovine bone (Bio-Oss®) eight months postoperative. Graft particles (violet) are included in newly formed bone.

reportedly considered to be the most physiological bone substitute; it becomes completely incorporated and integrated into the human bone after remodeling (Figs. 5.6 and 5.7).[57] Another commercially available product is Colloss®, a collagen type I lyophilisate in a triple helix structure (Ossacur GmbH, Oberstenfeld, Germany).

Disadvantages of deorganified bovine bone grafts are (besides their bovine origin) the increased risk of a host immune response, brittleness, easy migration, the recommendation to be combined with autogenous bone, and the mandatory use of GTR membranes with it.[43,45,58] Xenografts appear to incorporate into bone, but their slow resorption rates may have a negative impact on the quality of the newly formed bone and consequently on their clinical relevance. Public perception of the materials used as allografts and xenografts reduces the acceptance

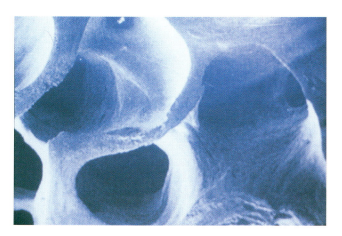

FIGURE 5.4. Three-dimensional architecture of human cancellous bone.

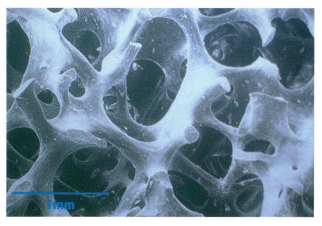

FIGURE 5.5. Figure clearly showing the same architecture in deorganified bovine bone (Bio-Oss®).

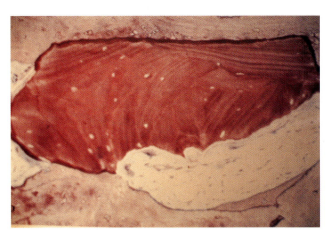

FIGURE 5.7. Magnification of a part of Figure 5.6 shows one particle that is part of the process of natural remodeling by osteoclasts (light).

of these materials. Furthermore, the potential for immunologic reactions can limit the use of these graft materials. The recent worldwide developments concerning bovine spongiform encephalopathy (BSE) disease strengthen the fear of disease transmission. BSE is not a disease caused by bacteria, fungi, or viruses; it is a prion disease. A prion is a modification of a protein into a prion-protein (PrPSc or proteinaceous infectious particle protein) that accumulates in the central nervous system and spleen. The outcome is inevitably lethal. To date, prions are highly resistant to all traditional chemical and physical procedures of inactivation, and no decontamination procedure existing today has been shown to be capable of inducing complete deactivation of the infectious agents, in spite of what manufacturers claim. In fact, these prions are not destroyed either by methods utilizing hot or cold treatments or by chemical or enzymatic methods. UV radiation, ionizing radiation, heat sterilization, and methods utilizing formaldehydes have also proven to be ineffective.[59–61] The acquired form of BSE disease in humans (CJD or Creutzfeld-Jacob Disease) can be transmitted by surgical instruments, EEG electrodes, grafts, or growth hormones and has been found in health care professionals such as neurosurgeons, dentists, nurses, and histopathologists. At the present time, there is no effective treatment or cure.[62,63]

Alloplasts

To avoid the previously mentioned complications and drawbacks of allografts and xenografts, biocompatible synthetic materials have been used over the past two decades. High expectations have been placed on their use in clinical applications, and recent advances have greatly improved their clinical outcome. They can be resorbable or nonresorbable; microporous (less than 350 μ), macro-

porous (greater than 350 μ), or nonporous; crystalline or amorphous; or granular or molded in form. There is a consensus about their advantages: they are readily available, sterile, easily stored, safe, and well tolerated. But their main advantage is the elimination of the possibility of cross-infection.

They are osteoconductive materials, but all differ from each other in some chemical and physical properties; these differing properties will determine which material is best for a specific clinical application.[43,64] There are three main groups of alloplasts:

1. Ceramics (synthetic hydroxyapatite, tricalcium phosphate, glass)
2. Calcium carbonate
3. Composite polymers (resorbable and nonresorbable)

CERAMICS

Synthetic Hydroxyapatite (HA)   Hydroxyapatite (HA), $Ca_{10}(PO_4)_6(OH)_2$, is the primary inorganic natural component of bone, comprising 60–70% of the calcified skeleton and 98% of dental enamel. It has a calcium to phosphorus ratio of 10:6. It is biocompatible and bonds readily to adjacent hard and soft tissues.[43,55,65] The clinical applications of this material are determined by the physical and chemical properties of the graft type used. The physical forms include porous (micro- or macro-) and nonporous forms, resorbable and nonresorbable forms, and blocks and particles. Chemical properties depend on the calcium to phosphorus ratio, the pH of the surrounding area, ionic substitution, and elemental impurities.[66] Large crystalline particles will take a very long time to resorb and are called nonresorbable; small-sized crystalline HA and amorphous HA will break down more quickly.[65] Therefore, the nature of the crystalline structure of the material determines the degree of resorption. On the other hand, porosity will determine the extent of blood permeability and vessel ingrowth into the graft. Pores of 250–350 μ are reported to be ideal for bone ingrowth. But unfortunately the strength decreases exponentially with the increase in porosity, which is considered a major disadvantage.[28,43–45,55] Solid, dense blocks have high compressive strength, but they are brittle, migrate under stress during the healing period, and are not suitable for load bearing. Strong and porous HA, with a compressive strength similar to that of bone, can be prepared in laboratories, but this material becomes clinically difficult to handle and contour. Currently available examples of this type of material are Calcitite® 2040 and 4060 (dense, nonresorbable particulates; Centerpulse, Dental Division, Carlsbad, California, U.S.A.); Osteograf/LD® (low density particles) and Osteograf/

D® (dense particles) (CeraMed Dental, Lakewood, Colorado, U.S.A.); Osteogen® (highly porous, resorbable particles; Impladent Ltd., Holliswood, New York, U.S.A.); and Orthomatrix® (dense, nonresorbable particles), which comes in 420–840 μ (HA-1000) and 250–420 μ (HA-500) sizes (Lifecore Biomedical, Chaska, Minnesota, U.S.A.). However, an important main disadvantage of these materials is that HA makes dental implant placement impossible or difficult to perform. The current use of HA as a grafting material is becoming limited, since it may be just an osseous defect filler (Figs. 5.8a,b and 5.9).

To overcome some of the material's difficult handling characteristics and physical properties, a combination product was developed: Hapset® (Lifecore Biomedical, Chaska, Minnesota, U.S.A.). It is 65% Orthomatrix® HA-500 and 35% calcium sulfate ($CaSO_4$) hemihydrate (medical-grade plaster of Paris). Dreesman, in 1892, reported the use of calcium sulfate in filling a variety of human osseous defects.[67] The calcium sulfate acts as a resorbable binder and helps to prevent the initial loss of HA particles. It is recommended that the surgical site be free of bleeding to promote initial hardening of the graft mass. The plaster resorbs within one month, leaving a scaffold of HA. The rationale for using medical-grade calcium sulfate is that (1) it acts as a barrier for three to four weeks, preventing undesirable soft tissue ingrowth, and (2) it helps to stabilize the bone graft, preventing excessive particle loss.[68] A controlled study of human periodontal defects filled with calcium sulfate alone showed no improvement over the controls.[69]

Tricalcium Phosphate (TCP) Tricalcium phosphate is chemically similar to HA, but it does not have the same chemical composition as natural bone. It has a calcium to phosphorus ratio of 3:2 and is converted partially into HA in the body.[70] Resorption rate is variable and is very dependent on the material's chemical structure. During the past few years, the α- and β-phases of TCP have been subjected to increasing attention. Variation of the sintering temperature allows the production of different crystalline phases. A temperature of 900°C allows the production of β-TCP; a further increase in temperature (greater than 1180°C) leads to a restructuring of the TCP to its α analogue. Alpha (α) or beta (β) refers to the particular orientation of the TCP crystals. Alpha-TCP resorbs very slowly and remains detectable in bone after many years, whereas β-TCP is fully resorbed and replaced by natural bone after eight to twelve months.[71] Clinical use of α-TCP is obviously not recommended, although there are such products commercially available (e.g., BioBvse®; BioVision, Freiburg, Germany). TCP thus provides a physical matrix suitable for the deposition of new bone, and

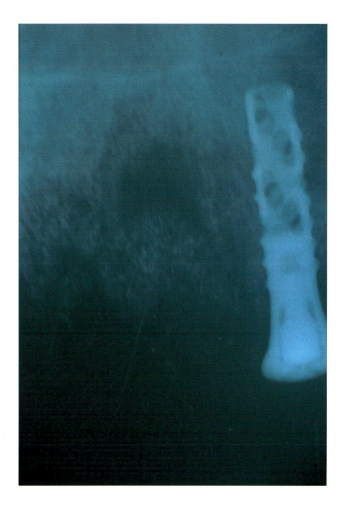

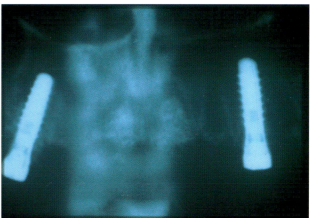

FIGURES 5.8a,b. These figures show the difficulty of completely filling extraction sockets with hydroxyapatite.

since the resorption rate of β-TCP is synchronous with the bone remodeling rate, one can expect full bone regeneration at the defect site, provided it is used in the proper clinical indication.[70,71] Note that the use of TCP is only

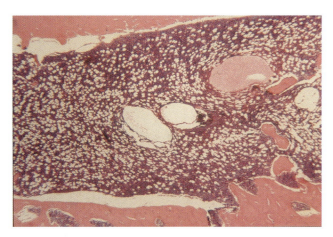

FIGURE 5.9. Figure showing the lack of integration between hydroxyapatite and host bone.

indicated for nonpathologic sites,[70,71] preferably combined with autogenous bone grafts or allografts (to improve its handling properties and osteoinductivity) and guided tissue regenerative techniques.[43] Commercially available TCP products include Augmen®, Synthograf®, Fortoss Resorb™, and Cerasorb® (Curasan Pharma GmbH, Kleinostheim, Germany) (Figs. 5.10 and 5.11).

Bioactive Glass   Bioactive glass grafts are a mixture of calcium salts and phosphate (in the same proportions as in bone and teeth), sodium salts, and silicon (which is essential for bone to mineralize). This mixture or composition is known as 45S5. The sizes of the granules vary between 90 and 710 μ, with an average of 300–355 μ. The material bonds to bone by forming a hydroxycarbonate apatite (HCA) layer on the surface of the glass,[72] closely imitating bone as a result of the incorporation of host material. A mechanically compliant collagen layer approximately 0.3 μ thick, which is very similar in dimensions to the natural periodontal ligament,[73,74] is created on the graft-bone interface; this is how this graft material is thought to help in the repair of ligaments. Bone transformation and regeneration occur within the hollow calcium phosphate chambers, at multiple sites, rapidly filling the defect with new bone that continuously remodels in its normal physiological manner.[73,75] This controlled bioactivity permits material transformation and bone remodeling to occur at the same time (Figs. 5.12 and 5.13). In an animal study[76] and another human study,[75] Schepers et al. reported that bioactive glass granules are easier to manipulate than HA granules and did not show any tendency to disperse into the surrounding tissues.[76] It formed a cohesive mass when contacting blood and did not float with bleeding. The possible differentiation of osteoprogenitor cells to osteoblasts might create an

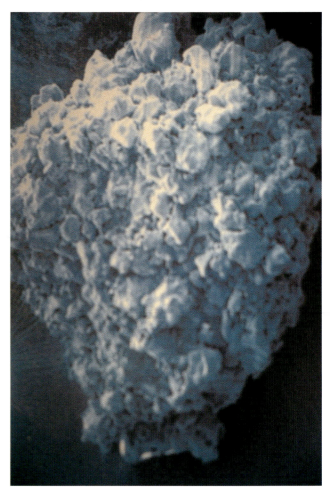

FIGURE 5.10.   One β-tricalcium phosphate particle of 200 μ (Cerasorb®).

enhanced prognosis, thus the graft will have an increased therapeutic effect.[40,41] However, other authors reported a rapid breakdown and loss of the graft material when it was exposed to oral fluids, with a very high risk for infection.[44,74] Commercially available products include Bioglass®, Perioglass® (U.S. Biomaterials, Baltimore, Maryland U.S.A.) and Biogran® (3i, Palm Beach Gardens, Florida, U.S.A.).

CALCIUM CARBONATE   The $CaCO_3$ graft material is made of aragonite (more than 98% $CaCO_3$), which is not altered by laboratory processing and has a porosity greater than 45%. The average pore size is 150 μ, and the granules are 300–450 μ and 630–1000 μ in diameter. The material resorbs slowly and needs no surface transformation to start the bone formation cascade: other materials must undergo a surface transformation, from HA to carbonate, but $CaCO_3$ apparently eliminates this step, which may permit more rapid bone formation at the grafting site.[77] Calcium carbon-

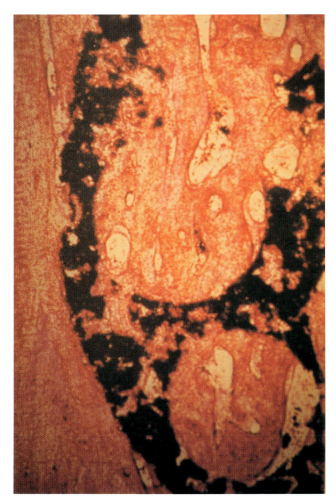

FIGURE 5.11. Newly formed bone (red) in and around the pores of the β-tricalcium phosphate graft (black), with simultaneous resorption of the graft.

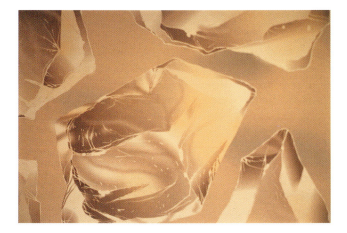

FIGURE 5.12. A 300–350 μ bioactive glass granule (Biogran®).

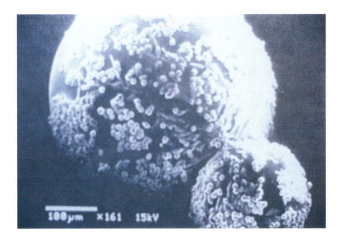

FIGURE 5.13. Calcium phosphate hollow chamber formed by phagocytes, where progenitor cells differentiate into osteoblasts.

under stress during the healing period.[44] The commercial available product is called Biocoral® (Inoteb s.a., Saint-Gonnéry, France).

COMPOSITE POLYMERS

Resorbable Synthetic biologically resorbable polymers have been known in medicine for a long time.[64] For many years products composed of either polylactic or polyglycolic acid have been used as a suture material, fixation screws, bone patches, and in many other clinical applications. Most of these polymers have a high molecular weight, yielding a breakdown time of up to three years, which is sometimes necessary for a particular clinical purpose, as in certain spinal column surgeries. Many factors play a role in the biological degradation of the polymers, including the age of the patient, the condition of the immune system, tissue tolerance, the location of the defect, and configuration of the exposed surface.[78] The final by-products of the enzymatic degradation of these polymers are carbon dioxide and water.[78] Recently, a low-density copolymer of polylactic acid and polyglycolic acid that permits an estimated degradation time of between a minimum of three to four months and a maximum of six to eight months was made available in three different forms (powder, sponge, and gel) that can be combined to permit the filling of every possible type of bone defect. The powder is more indicated for three-wall osseous defects, the sponge for two- or three-wall defects; they are dampened slightly with physiological solution or the patient's own blood and formed into the correct shape by a scalpel or any sharp instrument prior to insertion. The gel can be used for deep defects, where it is "injected" directly via a syringe. The small mass and large surface

ate grafts appear to have good hemostatic properties and are not readily displaced from the treatment site. However, this material is also brittle and migrates area of this graft material permits the fibroblasts to easily penetrate into it and initiate absorption and cell colonization. This graft material is easy to work with. It is commercially available as Fisiograft® (GHIMAS spa. Bolognia, Italy). However, the use of guided tissue regenerative barriers is often necessary. Histological findings seem very promising, but all data are very recent and available clinical follow-up is only within a few months.

Nonresorbable This bone alloplast material is a patented nonresorbable chemically pure mixture of polymethylmethacrylate (PMMA) and polyhydroxylethylmethacrylate (PHEMA), with small amounts of barium sulfate for radiopacity and an outer surface of calcium hydroxide graft material, which makes the direct interface with the host bone and forms $CaCO_3$ apatite in the presence of the bleeding marrow. Since the polymerization reaction occurs in the laboratory, there is no heat generated to the tissues and no chance of monomer contamination: these two important side effects are totally eliminated.

PMMA is a synthetic polymer used extensively for years in a variety of implantable and other medical devices, including intraocular lenses, prosthetic heart valves, reconstructive prosthetic dental devices; in cranioplasty implants; and to encase intracranial aneurysms. The first inner layer is coated with a layer of PHEMA, a hydrophilic polymer that also has an extensive history of use in medical devices, for example, contact lenses and burn dressings (Hydron®). The material has a unique hollow, spherical architecture with a pore size opening of approximately 350 μ and a particle size of 750 μ, which allows bone growth into and around the material and creates a matrix with increased surface area and greater ingrowth possibilities. Following healing, only 10–12% of the volume fill of a defect consists of this graft material, while 88–90% is regenerating, remodeling bone.[79]

The synergy of graft components results in unique properties and physical characteristics. The most important and unique characteristic of the material is its negatively charged surface (–10 mV). Wolff showed that such a negative surface charge facilitates and enhances bone healing and bone formation.[80] Studies on salamanders proved that they use an extremely weak current to regenerate completely lost body parts.[81] When the same negative charge is used in bone diseases (e.g., osteomyelitis), healing of the bone occurs.[81] Although the material is neither bacteriostatic nor even bactericidal, bacteria do not easily colonize on the surface of the polymer because both the material and bacteria have a negative surface charge; thus, the material might impede the devolopment of infection.[81] This negative charge also allows the polymer to adhere to bone (because of the positively charged cells); to attract the pluripotential precursor cells that will

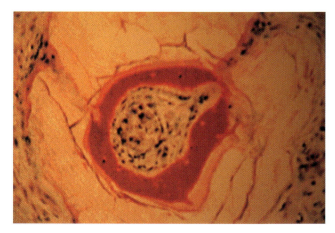

FIGURE 5.14. Precursor cells are attracted immediately to the surface of a nonresorbable copolymer particle (Bioplant HTR®).

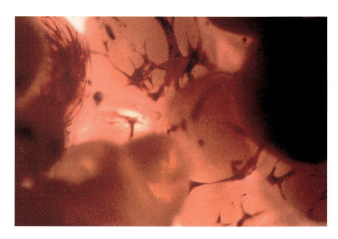

FIGURE 5.15. Intimate contact and immediate proliferation of precursor cells on the surface of the graft due to its negative (–10 mV) charge.

form osteoblasts on its surface (Figs. 5.14 and 5.15); and to adhere to metal[82] (Fig. 5.16), enhancing osseointegration (Fig. 5.17) around metal implants.[79,83–85] Furthermore, the material does not undergo any migration under loads. Most of the commercially available bone grafting materials require GTR membranes for ensuring predictable results,[84,85] but with the use of this material, the need for the membrane may be eliminated, because it is claimed that the material itself acts as a membrane. The nonresorbable polymer material, when wetted with bleeding marrow, initially forms dense fibrous tissue under the mucosal flap and develops a substantial compressive strength (up to 1800 psi).[79,83–85]

In animal studies, new bone, PDL, and new cementum were formed around and in the material. Sharpey's fibers also were observed without other intervening tissues.[86] And in human studies, an author reported a 65% regen-

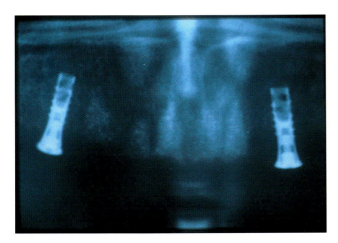

FIGURE 5.16. A 100% fill of every extraction socket.

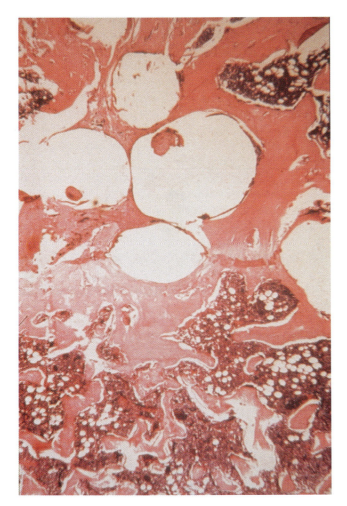

FIGURE 5.17. Complete integration of grafting material and newly formed bone.

eration rate for new cementum, new bone, and normal PDL.[55] A possibility of slow material resorption (twelve years) also was reported.[86] The material can be applied regularly in all intraoral grafting procedures.[84,85,87] The commercially available product is called Bioplant HTR® (Bioplant, Inc., South Norwalk, Connecticut, U.S.A.)

REGENERATIVE BARRIERS

Barrier membranes were first tested in the late 1950s for the healing of cortical defects in orthopedic research and were first described by Hurley et al.[88] However, this pioneer study did not lead to broad clinical applications of the membrane techniques for similar defects. Nyman et al., who examined barrier membranes in periodontal wound regeneration in the early 1980s,[89] recognized the potential of this technique. The barrier is basically used to prevent invasion of competing soft tissue cells from the overlying mucosa.

Critical work by Karring et al. and Buser et al.[90,91] has explored different membrane devices that separate tissues during healing. This technology has been termed guided bone regeneration (GBR). The principles of GBR are derived from the knowledge generated by guided tissue regeneration (GTR). GBR shares with GTR the use of barrier membranes to achieve regeneration of new tissues. But where the goal of GTR is to regenerate bone, cementum, new attachment, and periodontal ligament contiguous with root structure(s), the only goal of GBR is to regenerate bone.[92] It seems reasonable to assume that GBR procedures are even more predictable than GTR procedures for osseous regeneration, because the regeneration in GTR occurs in a hostile healing environment due to the proximity of root surfaces contaminated with plaque, calculus, and toxins. This hostile environment is contrary to the situation in GBR procedures. Additional use of bone-grafting materials for space maintenance tends to improve GBR outcomes.[93] GBR today is a widely accepted regenerative treatment modality in the implant dentistry. Guided bone regenerative membranes are used to

- Separate tissues during healing,
- Retard apical migration of epithelium to the site,
- Maintain the necessary space for bone ingrowth (tenting), and
- Protect the graft material in the defect.[92]

GBR barriers are of two types, nonresorbable and resorbable.

Nonresorbable

EXPANDED POLYTETRAFLUOROETHYLENE
Expanded polytetrafluoroethylene (ePTFE) is sintered, and has pores between 5 and 30 μ in the structure of the material itself. The most popular commercial type is

Gore-Tex® (W. L. Gore & Assoc., Flagstaff, Arizona, U.S.A.).

NANO POLYTETRAFLUOROETHYLENE (NPTFE)

With nano polytetrafluoroethylene (nPTFE), there is no sintering, making the material quite pliable, allowing easier tenting and adaptation; the pores are between 0.2 and 0.3 μ, and the smaller pore size is believed to limit epithelial ingrowth and bacterial infiltration.[94] Commercially available products are TefGen-FD and TefGen-Plus (Lifecore Biomedical, Chaska, Minnesota, U.S.A.).

TITANIUM Most of the membranes are made of titanium foil with micropores (e.g., Frios® BoneShield, and JMP Titanium Mesh™; Friadent GmbH, Mannheim, Germany). Sometimes the surface is also treated to attain a titanium oxide surface (e.g., Ti TitaniumOxid Mesh).

COMBINATION Sometimes ePTFE membranes are reinforced with titanium, for example, Gore-Tex® Titanium Reinforced (W. L. Gore & Assoc., Flagstaff, Arizona, U.S.A.).

The major disadvantage of these types of nonresorbable membranes is the need for a second surgical procedure to remove them. This second surgery can sometimes be a tedious undertaking and can also disturb healing and soft tissue integrity.[95] Patients today are not eager to accept this type of treatment.[95] Another disadvantage is that membrane exposure rates of up to 31%,[96] caused by flap sloughing or incision-line opening, have been the cause of postsurgical complications and failures. Membrane exposure provides a channel of communication between the oral environment and newly forming tissues, increasing the chance for infection and decreasing bone regeneration potential. These disadvantages and other minor problems led to the development of resorbable barriers.

Resorbable

NATURAL

- Polylactic and citric acid ester (resorption time eight to ten weeks): Guidor® (Butler, Chicago, Illinois, U.S.A.).
- Glycolate and lactate polymers (resorption time ten weeks): Vicryl-mesh™ (Johnson & Johnson, Sommerville, New Jersey, U.S.A.).
- Glycolate and lactate polymers, arranged in a random fiber, trilayer matrix lacking large holes (resorption time ten weeks): Gore Resolut XT™ (W. L. Gore & Assoc., Flagstaff, Arizona, U.S.A.).
- Polyglycolic acid, polylactic acid, trimethylene carbonate (resorption time twelve to fourteen months): Gore Osseoquest (W. L. Gore & Assoc., Flagstaff, Arizona, U.S.A.).
- Bovine Achilles tendon collagen: BioMend™ (resorption time six to eight weeks) or BioMend™ Extend

(resorption time fifteen to eighteen weeks) (Centerpulse, Dental Division , Carlsbad, California, U.S.A.).
- Bovine collagen tendon (resorption time sixteen to twenty-four weeks): BioSorb® (Imtec Corp, Ardmore, Oklahoma, U.S.A.).
- Bilayer collagen from pigs (resorption time six to eight months): Bio-Gide® and Perio- Gide® (Geistlich Pharma AG, Wolhusen, Swizerland).
- Collagen from porcine dermis (resorption time four months): AlloDerm® P (Lifecell Corp., Branchburg, New Jersey, U.S.A.)
- Collagen from human dermis (resorption time four months): AlloDerm® H. (Lifecell Corp., Branchburg, New Jersey, U.S.A.). Donated human skin is aseptically processed to become a framework without any human cells, creating an acellular, biocompatible human connective tissue matrix.

Collagen membranes have become the subject of research lately, mainly because of their favorable biological properties.[97] Type I collagen is a predominant component found in periodontal connective tissue and forms the main component of this type of membrane (Bio-Gide® has types I and III). In addition, collagen possesses extra advantages, including weak immunogenicity, hemostasis, and chemotaxis for fibroblasts.[97] When implanted into the body, collagen is absorbed at a rate that can be controlled by the degree of chemical treatment or cross-linkage. Various cross-linking techniques have been developed, such as ultraviolet light, hexamethylenediisocyanate(HMDIC), diphenylphosphorylazide (DPPA), and glutaraldehyde (GA) or formaldehyde (FA) plus irradiation. But cross-linkage seems to inhibit epithelial migration effectivly.[97]

In conclusion products that resorb very slowly seem to favor bone-grafting success.

SYNTHETIC

- Poly DL-lactide dissolved in N-methyl-2-pyrrolidone. This material is commercially obtained as a liquid that sets to a firm consistency when contacted with water or other aqueous solutions. It can be shaped extraorally and adheres to the defect without sutures. Resorption time is twelve months, and the commercial name is Atrisorb® (Atrix Labs, Fort Collins, Colorado, U.S.A.).
- Calcium sulfate (plaster of Paris). As stated earlier, $CaSO_4$ has been used since 1892.[67] This material (Fortoss Cema™, Capset®; Lifecore Biomedical, Chaska, Minnesota, U.S.A.) is mixed and then placed over the graft material. Resorption time is four weeks.

Although GBR membranes are a widely accepted treatment modality, their clinical application should be approached with caution. In many instances, they showed compromised wound closure, with the risk of membrane exposure and bacterial infiltration, either due to clinical mishandling or unknown reasons.

When resorbable membranes are used, degradation occurs mostly via hydrolysis. This creates an acid environment, which can have a negative effect on bone formation.[92,96,97] Only collagen membranes seem to be absorbed through catabolic processes resembling those involved in normal tissue turnover.[67] On the other hand, an animal study reported the fast degradation of three types of collagen membranes (BioGide, AlloDerm porcine-derived, and AlloDerm human-derived) that puts in question the effectiveness of these types of resorbable membranes when they are to be used as physical barriers beyond one month.[98]

CYTOKINES

Levander made one of the earliest suggestions of the presence of protein extracts that induce new bone formation when implanted subcutaneously or intramuscularly.[99] He proposed that the implanted bone material contains soluble stimulating agents that promote new bone formation. Lacroix confirmed these findings by showing that an alcoholic extract of bone cartilaginous epiphyses promoted bone formation. He termed this substance *osteogenin*.[100] Urist, in 1965, observed that protein extracts could induce the local formation of new cartilage and bone when implanted at nonbony sites. He later showed that protein extracts from decalcified bone matrix were responsible for new bone formation and could be separated.[101] However, clinical application was very restricted because of the difficulty of the extraction process. The advent of molecular biology and, in particular, recombinant DNA technology permitted the production of relatively large quantities of these proteins.

The family name of all these proteins is cytokines; these can be divided into two major categories: growth factors (GFs) and bone morphogenetic proteins (BMPs). Their activity is significantly different: GFs cause several general activities, whereas BMPs focus only on differentiating cells.[47,102] GFs also change the growth rate of preexisting bone, while BMPs induce new bone formation limited to the site of implantation.

Growth Factors

The available growth factors types are

• Transforming growth factor beta (TGF-β),
• Insulinlike growth factors I and II (IGF-I; IGF-II),
• Fibroblast growth Factor (FGF),
• Epidermal growth factor (EGF), and
• Platelet derived growth factor (PDGF).

All growth factor types modulate healing events by stimulating the migration and proliferation of a broad range of mesenchymal cells.[103] They also stimulate osteoblast-like cells to proliferate and synthesize collagen. This is the rationale behind the new commercially available platelet rich plasma (PRP). Platelets or thrombocytes contain numerous GFs that are released during the natural healing process.[104] The growth of new blood vessels (angiogenesis), especially, is stimulated through PRP, and this is the first and most important step towards rebuilding the defect area. The use of the patient's own PRP seems to improve the safety and quality of the newly formed bone.[104] Usually, PRP is produced by the techniques of "plasmapheresis" or "thrombopheresis" via a centrifuge collection system. PRP is prepared from just half a liter of the patient's own blood. It has to be considered that the activity of platelets rapidly decreases after harvesting, so the period of time between harvesting and the clinical use of the PRP has to be kept as short as possible (maximum forty-five minutes). However, most of the growth factors including PRP seem to be more active in the soft tissue regeneration as well as in bone formation. Therefore, research must be directed toward developing site-specific effects. Today, PRP concentrate can be advantageous for patients with reduced wound healing.[104] New technology has recently been introduced by Harvest® SmartPReP™ (Harvest Technologies Corp., Plymouth, MA, U.S.A.) to produce a bioactive platelet gel called "SmartClot™." It provides a revolutionary platelet-harvesting process while preserving platelet viability with its bioactive properties.

Bone Morphogenetic Proteins

Actually, more than twenty structurally unique BMPs have been identified, all of which can produce ectopic bone formation.[48] The advent of molecular biology techniques and, in particular, recombinant DNA technology has substantially increased the possibility of producing relatively large quantities of these proteins.[47] The use of recombinant BMP offers some critical advantages over the use of BMPs derived from human cadaver bones: there are no contaminating proteins and no risk of transmitting infectious disease. Thirteen proteins have already been purified and cloned; they are called BMP-1 through BMP-13.[47] One of these, recombinant human BMP-2 (rhBMP-2), has been assayed in several systems and has been found to have very high osteogenic activity, making rhBMP-2 most promising.[48,49,105] BMPs induce formation of new bone that has all the characteristics of normal bone, including cartilage formation followed by endochondral ossification. BMPs accelerate the time of implant-bone integration and have excellent therapeutic potential in dental and periodontal attachment complex repair.[49,105] However, they are all highly active, which leaves the question still unanswered of how to control their activity. The full potential and safety of BMPs will require further clinical studies.

How to deliver cytokines to the graft site still remains debatable. All need an appropriate carrier for regular clinical use. The ideal carrier must maximize host tissue exposure to the cytokines and ensure uniform delivery without allowing spread of the substance beyond the boundaries of the graft site. The carrier should be safe and biocompatible. Several carriers have been tested, and from the latest results it seems that synthetic polymers may prove to be a reasonable carrier.[47,49]

DISTRACTION OSTEOGENESIS

Besides conventional bone grafting methods to treat the lack of bone, distraction osteogenesis can become a viable alternative.[106] The technique is based on the "floating bone principle": the natural tendency of fractured bone to bridge defects by immediate callus formation.[107] A directed distraction of the fracture ends by means of microplates (distractors) will activate bone growth to fill up the gap. The distracters are made exclusively of pure titanium and carry a slide mechanism with attached microplates. Following adjustment of the microplates, the buccocortical osteotomy is performed to mobilize an adequate section of the alveolar crest.. The distraction is then carried out, one week after the surgery, by activating the device about 1 mm a day (0.5 mm, two times) until the desired gain in height is obtained. Following the dis-

traction phase, a retention or consolidation period of three months must be observed. The average gain in vertical height after a completed treatment can reach up to 10.2 mm (Figs. 5.18–5.20). Implants can then be inserted. This procedure gains a time advantage of approximately nine weeks over the conventional augmenting techniques, where a consolidation of at least six months is required. Contraindications to this type of treatment are in general the same as for implant treatment (bone diseases, radiotherapy of greater than 60 Gy, smoking habits, etc.) and include negative perception by the patient; however, a specific contraindication is a starting height of less than 6 mm of remaining bone, due to the high risk of jaw fracture.[108–110]

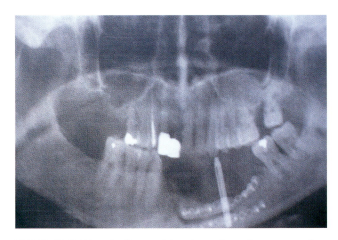

FIGURE 5.19. Radiographic view after placement of the distractor.

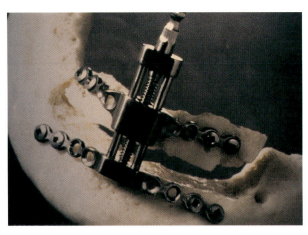

FIGURE 5.18. Distraction device (TRACK 1.5, Tissue Regeneration by Alveolar Callus distraction Köln).

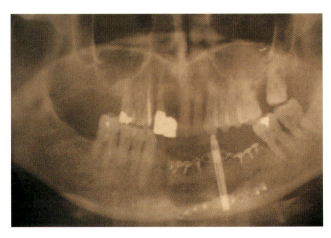

FIGURE 5.20. Radiographic view at the end of the distraction phase, showing approximately 12 mm of bone height gained.

TITANIUM MESH

Severe alveolar bone resorption can sometimes be a clinical dilemma that impairs optimal implant placement in the alveolar ridge; it mandates particular bone-grafting procedures that can offer predictable results. Autogenous corticotrabicular grafts used in treating severe osseous defects have clinical short comings: the blood supply to the graft can be minimized (especially when using large grafts),[111] there is an increased risk of surgical morbidity, and the graft may lose 30% or more of its overall size due to postoperative bone remodeling.[30,112] Guided bone regenerative membranes can help in treating larger vertical osseous defects, but the inherited physical property of the membrane to collapse towards the defect due to the pressure of the overlying soft tissues (thus reducing the space required for regeneration) makes the overall amount of regenerated bone questionable. The physical characteristics of the GBR membranes could be improved by the application of titanium strips. This procedure allows the preservation of the space for regeneration by what is called tenting. [9]

The use of titanium mesh can be a predicable and reliable treatment modality for regenerating and reconstructing a severely deficient alveolar ridge.[10,113–118] A study[118] that involved the use of a titanium mesh to protect the regenerating tissues and to achieve a rigid fixation of autogenous bone segments was conducted with twenty-five patients. It concluded that the use of titanium mesh can assist bone regeneration in non-space-making defects, since it probably does not interfere with the blood flow to the underlying tissues because of the presence of microholes within the mesh. The study also confirmed that the quantity of bone regenerated under the membranes is directly related to the amount of space present underneath. The main advantages of the titanium mesh are that it maintains and preserves the space to be regenerated without being collapsed or bent, it provides blood supply for the bone-grafting material directly from the periosteum through its micropores, and it is completely biocompatible to oral tissues.[119]

The preoperative steps for using the titanium mesh entail a thorough presurgical planning,[120] which includes a proper assessment of the size and nature of the osseous defect[121] and making preoperative working casts for tailing and fitting the titanium mesh sheet to the space of the osseous defect (Figs. 5.21a–d and 5.22a–d). The intraoperative steps involve a midcrestal incision extended mesially and distally beyond the area to be grafted. Another two vertical incisions are made at both ends of the crestal incision on the buccal side, with complete mucoperiosteal flap mobilization. The osseous defect is decorticated to enhance the cellular flow to the graft. The placement of the titanium mesh requires sequential placement steps: first the palatal side of the mesh (Mondeal Medical Systems GmbH, Tuttlingen, Germany) is fixed in place and tightened with two microscrews), then another two screw holes are drilled in the labial side in the cortical bone and marked with the naked eye in order to not lose their original place.

The grafting material is prepared and introduced to the area of the defect (the preferred grafting material is particulated bone marrow with allogenous bone particles), and the space is overfilled (Fig. 5.23a–f). The titanium mesh is then laid to the labial side and fixed to the

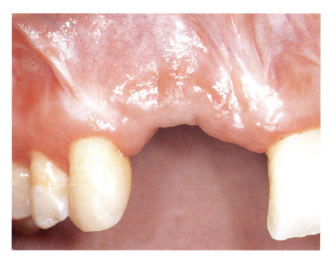

FIGURE 5.21a. Preoperative view of a forty-five-year-old woman showing excessive bone loss in both vertical and horizontal dimensions.

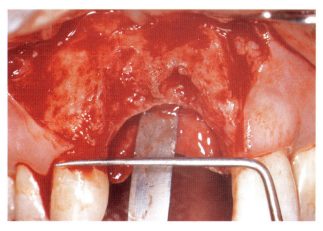

FIGURE 5.21b. Intraoperative view showing a 6 mm osseous defect.

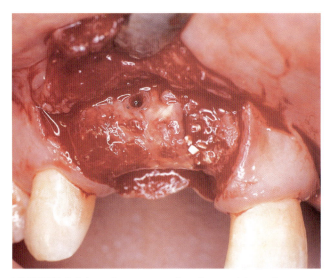

FIGURE 5.21c. Seven months after grafting, view showing the complete bone regeneration in the area using the titanium mesh.

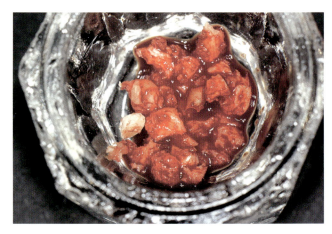

FIGURE 5.22b. Autogenous bone chips harvested from the chin to be particulated with the allogenous graft particles.

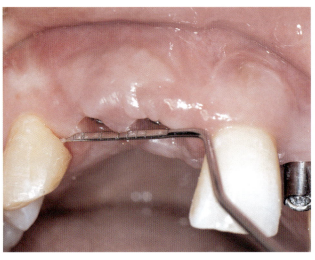

FIGURE 5.21d. Six weeks after abutment connection, showing remarkable improvement of the papillary height.

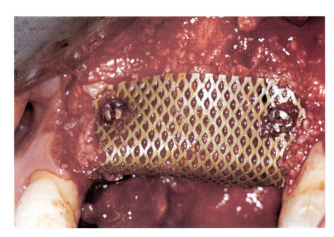

FIGURE 5.22c. The titanium mesh (Mondeal Medical Systems GMBH, Tuttlingen, Germany) fixed in place with the bone graft placed underneath.

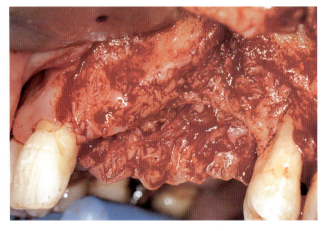

FIGURE 5.22a. Preoperative view of severe alveolar ridge resorption.

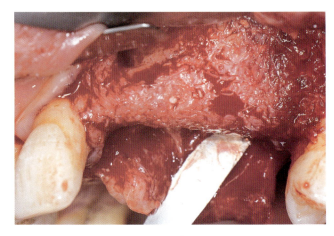

FIGURE 5.22d. Seven months postoperative view showing improved bone topography.

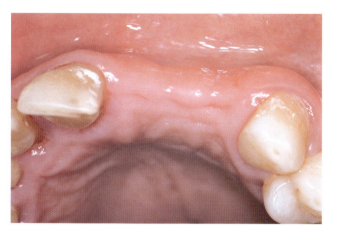

FIGURE 5.23a. A fifty-two-year-old man with missing maxillary right central and lateral incisors.

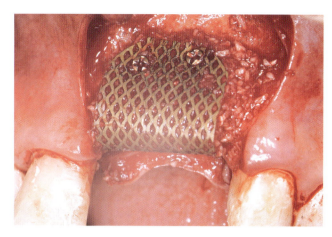

FIGURE 5.23d. The labial end of the mesh is stabilized to the labial plate. Note the sequential steps of the mesh fixation.

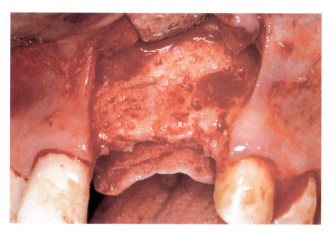

FIGURE 5.23b. The area after flap reflection showing severe bone loss in the horizontal plane. Note that the labial plate is being decorticated.

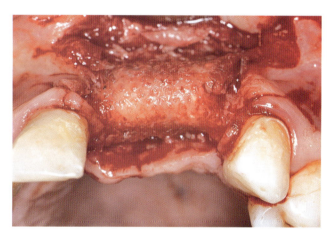

FIGURE 5.23e. Seven months postoperative view showing the regenerated bone after removal of the mesh.

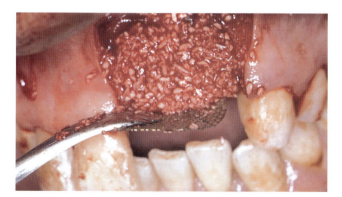

FIGURE 5.23c. The titanium mesh being stabilized palatally with two micro fixation screws (Mondeal Medical Systems GMBH, Tuttlingen, Germany).The particulated bone-grafting mix is introduced to the site (human allograft bone tissue, Allosource, Denver, Colorado). Note the sequential steps of the mesh fixation.

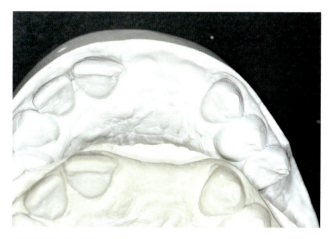

FIGURE 5.23f. Post- and preoperative models showing the improvement of the osseous topography after the treatment.

labial plate with the microscrews and tightened to its previously prepared place. Care should be exersised to not expose the margins of the titanium mesh through the margins of the mucoperiosteal flap. The importance of the sequence in stabilizing the mesh is that it saves the particulate bone graft from being dispersed or displaced during the drilling procedure for making the labial screw holes.

Optimal soft tissue closure on top of the titanium mesh is a vital clinical step that contributes to the success of the grafting procedure, because any opening of the incision line can jeopardize graft success.[122] (Refer to the method of soft tissue closure in critical conditions in Chapter 4).

Titanium mesh can be used before placing dental implants (staged approach) or in conjunction with dental implant placement (nonstaged approach). The choice depends primarily on the amount of bone available to stabilize the implant (Figure 5.24a–d).

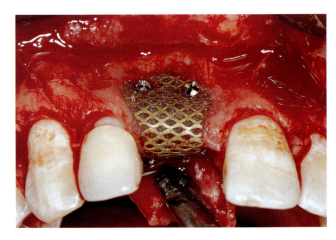

FIGURE 5.24c.   The titanium mesh (Modeal Medical Systems GMBH, Tuttlingen, Germany) stabilized in place, protecting the bone graft.

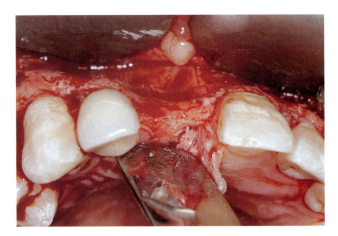

FIGURE 5.24a.   Intraoperative view of a thirty-year-old patient with missing right central incisor with the mucoperiosteal flap reflected, showing horizontal bone loss.

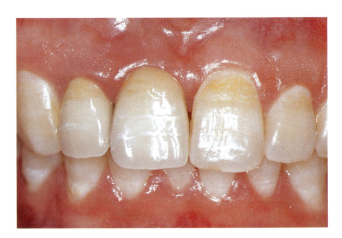

FIGURE 5.24d.   The case finally restored; note the improved profile.

CONCLUSION

The decision to use any particular grafting material or grafting technique should be based on the

- Nature and size of the defect,
- Physical properties of the graft,
- Chemical properties of the graft,
- Mechanism(s) of action of the graft,
- Assumed rehabilitation planning, and
- Required final result.

Today's practitioner has a wide array of grafting materials available that can be used in several clincal applications. The use of these materials has widened tremendously the scope and expectations for implant surgery. Research and clinical experience have shown

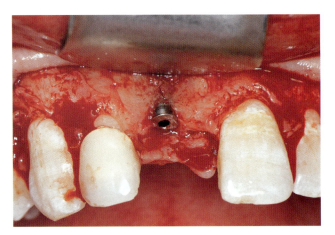

FIGURE 5.24b.   The implant placement (TSV Paragon, Centerpulse, Dental Division, Carlsbad, California). Labial dehiscence occurred to reduced bone width.

that certain materials are better suited for specific applications than others and are much easier to handle than others. Keeping this in mind, the clinician must give priority to thorough presurgical planning and to considering less invasive procedures that attain predictable results.

REFERENCES

1. Johnson K. A study of the dimensional changes occurring in the maxilla after tooth extraction. Part I: Normal healing. Aust Dent J 1963(8): 428–433.

2. Carlsson GE, Bergman B, and Headegard B. Changes in contour of the maxillary alveolar process under immediate dentures. A longitudinal clinical and x-ray cephalometric study covering 5 years. Acta Odontol Scand 1967(25): 45–75.

3. Jovanovic SA. Bone rehabilitation to achieve optimal aesthetics. Pract Periodont Aesthet Dent 1997(9): 41–52.

4. Jovanovic SA, Paul SJ, and Nishimura R D. Anterior implant-supported reconstructions: A surgical challenge. Pract Periodont Aesthet Dent 1999(11): 551–558.

5. Salama H, Salama MA, Garber D, and Adar P. The interproximal height of bone: A guidepost to predictable aesthetic strategies and soft tissue contours in anterior tooth replacement. Pract Periodont Aesthet Dent 1998(10): 1131–1142.

6. Dooren EV. Management of soft and hard tissue surrounding dental implants: Aesthetic principles. Pract Periodont Aesthet Dent 2000(12): 837–841.

7. Buser D, Dula K, Hirt HP, et al. Lateral ridge augmentation using autografts and barrier membranes: A clinical study with 40 partially edentulous patients. J Oral Maxillofac Surg 1996(54): 420–433.

8. Javanovic SA, Spiekermann H, and Richter EJ. Bone regeneration on titanium dental implants with dehisced defect sites. A clinical study. Int J Oral Maxillofac Implants 1992(7): 233–245.

9. Simion M, Jovanovic S, Trisi P, et al. Vertical ridge augmentation around dental implants using a membrane technique and autogenous bone or allografts in humans. Int J Periodont Rest Dent 1998(18): 8–23.

10. Sumi Y, Miyaishi O, Tohnai I, and Ueda M. Alveolar ridge augmentation with titanium mesh and autogenous bone. Oral Surg Oral Med Oral Pathol Oral Radiol Endod 2000(89): 268–270.

11. El Askary AS and Pipco DJ. Autogenous and allogenous bone grafting techniques to maximize esthetics. J Prosthet Dent 2000(83): 153–157.

12. Boyne PJ. Use of carrier materials in delivery of bone inductor substances. In Wise DL, ed. Biomaterials Engineering and Devices: Human Application, vol. 1. Totowa, NJ: Humana Press, Inc., 2000, 251–265.

13. Boyne PJ. Maxillofacial surgical application of bone inductor materials. Implant Dent 2000(10): 2–4.

14. Boyne PJ, Nakamura A, and Shabahang S. Evaluation of the long-term effect of function on rhBMP-2 regenerated hemimandibulectomy defects. Br J Oral Maxillofac Surg 1999(37): 344–352.

15. Hanada K, Dennis JE, and Caplan AL. Stimulatory effects of basic fibroblast growth factor and bone morphogenetic protein-2 on osteogenic differentiation of rat bone marrow-derived mesenchymal stem cells. J Bone Miner Res 1997(12): 1606–1614.

16. Meffert R. Guided tissue regeneration/guided bone regeneration: A review of the barrier membranes. Pract Periodont Aesthect Dent 1986(8): 142–148.

17. Laurell L and Gottlow J. Guided tissue regeneration update. Int Dent J 1998 48(Aug.): 386–398.

18. Lundgren AK, Lundgren D, Sennerby L, Taylor A, Gottlow J, and Nyman S. Bone augmentation at titanium implants using autologous bone grafts and a bioresorbable barrier. An experimental study in the rabbit tibia. Clin Oral Implant Res 1997(8): 82–89.

19. Lundgren D, Laurell L, Gottlow J, Rylander H, Mathisen T, Nyman S, and Rask M. The influence of the design of two different bioresorbable barriers on the results of guided tissue regeneration therapy. An intra-individual comparative study in the monkey. J Periodontol 1995(66): 605–612.

20. Gottlow J. Guided tissue regeneration using bioresorbable and non-resorbable devices: initial healing and long-term results, J Periodontol 1993(64): 1157–1165.

21. Yukna CN and Yukna RA. Multi-center evaluation of bioabsorbable collagen membrane for guided tissue regeneration in human Class II furcations. J Periodontol 1996(67): 650–657.

22. Becker W, Dahlin C, Lekholm U, Bergstrom C, van Steenberghe D, Higuchi K, and Becker BE. Five-year evaluation of implants placed at extraction and with dehiscences and fenestration defects augmented with ePTFE membranes: Results from a prospective multicenter study. Clin Implant Dent Relat Res 1999(1): 27–32.

23. Fiorellini JP, Engebretson SP, Donath K, and Weber HP. Guided bone regeneration utilizing expanded polytetrafluoroethylene membranes in combination with submerged and nonsubmerged dental implants in beagle dogs. J Periodontol 1998(69): 528–535.

24. Shanaman RH. A retrospective study of 237 sites treated consecutively with guided tissue regeneration. Int J Periodontics Restorative Dent 1994(14): 292–301.

25. Roccuzzo M, Lungo M, Corrente G, and Gandolfo S. Comparative study of a bioresorbable and non-resorbable membrane in the treatment of human buccal gingival recessions. J Periodontol 1996(67): 7–14

26. Hardwick R, Hayes BK, and Flynn C. Devices for dentoalveolar regeneration: An up-to-date literature review, J Periodontol 1995(66): 495–505.

27. Schwartz A, Melloing J, Carnes D, de la Fontaine J, Cochran D, Dean D, and Boyan B. Ability of commercial de-mineralized freeze-dried bone allograft to induce new bone formation. J Periodontol 1996(67): 918–926.

28. Burchardt H. Biology of bone transplantation. Orthop Clin North Am 1987(18): 187–195.

29. Sindet-Pedersen S, and Enemark H. Reconstruction of alveolar clefts with mandibular or iliac crest bone grafts: A comparative study. J Oral Maxillofac Surg 1990(48): 554–558.

30. Misch C. Ridge augmentation using mandibular ramus bone grafts for the placement of dental implants: Presentation of a technique. Pract Periodont Aesthet Dent 1996(8): 127–135.

31. Becker W, Clokie C, Sennerby L, Urist M, and Becker B. Histologic finding after implantation, an evaluation of different grafting materials and titanium micro screws in extraction sockets: Case reports. J Periodontol 1998(69): 414–421.

32. Hunt DR and Jovanovic SA. Autogenous bone harvesting: A chin graft technique for particulate and monocortical bone blocks. Int J Periodontics Restorative Dent 1999(19): 165–173.

33. Kalk W, Raghoebari G, Jansma J, and Boering G. Morbidity from iliac crest bone harvesting. J Oral Maxillofac Surg 1996(54): 1424–1429.

34. Hoppenreijs T, Nijdam E, and Freihofer H. The chin as a donor site in early secondary osteoplasty: A retrospective clinical and radiological evaluation. J Craniomaxillofac Surg 1992(20): 119–124.

35. Chin M and Toth BA. Distraction osseogenesis in maxillofacial surgery using internal devices: Review of five cases. J Oral Maxillofac Surg 1996(45): 45–52.

36. Gaggl A, Scultes G, and Karcher H. Vertical alveolar ridge distraction with prosthetic treatable distractors: A clinical investigation. Int J Oral Maxillofac Implants 2000 15(5): 701–710.

37. Hidding J, Lazar F, and Zöller JE. The vertical distraction of the alveolar bone. J Craniomaxillofac Surg 1998(26): 72–76.

38. Gaggl A, Schultes G, and Kärcher H. Distraction implants—A new possibility for the augmentative treatment of the edentulous atrophic mandible: Case report. Br J Oral Maxillofac Surg 1999(37): 481–485.

39. Skouteris CA and Sotereanos GC. Donor site morbidity following harvesting of autogenous rib grafts. J Oral Maxillofac Surg 1989(47): 808–812.

40. Williams DF. Bone healing processes. J Bio Eng 1987(1): 231–245.

41. Kenley R, Marden L, Turek T, Jin L, Ron E, and Hollinger JO. Osseous regeneration. J Biomed Mater Res 1994(28): 1139–1147.

42. Bao JY. Comparative bone healing. J Biomater Sci Polym 1997(8): 517–532

43. Misch CE and Dietsh F. Bone-grafting materials in implant dentistry. Implant Dent 1993(2): 158–167.

44. Gross JS. Bone grafting materials for dental applications: A practical guide. Compend Cont Educ Dent 1997(18): 1013–1038.

45. Lane JM. Bone graft substitutes. West J Med 1995(163): 565–567.

46. Tatum OJ, Jr. Osseous grafts in intra-oral sites. J Oral Implant 1996(22): 51–52.

47. Barboza E, Caula A, and Machado F. Potential of recombinant human bone morphogenetic protein-2 in bone regeneration. Implant Dent 1999(4): 360–366.

48. Wang EA, Rosen V, D'Alessandro JS, et al. Recombinant human bone morphogenetic protein induces bone formation. Proc Natl Acad Sci USA 1990(87): 2220–2224.

49. Toriumi DM, Kotler HS, Luxenberg DP, et al. Mandibular reconstruction with a recombinant bone-inducing factor: Functional, histologic and biomechanical evaluation. Arch Otolaryngol Head Neck Surg 1991(117): 1101–1112.

50. Rummelhart JM, Mellonig JT, Gray JL, et al. Bone allografts in periodontal therapy. J. Periodontol 1989(60): 655–663.

51. Second-hand Bones? (editorial) Lancet 1992(340): 1443.

52. Pinholt EM, Haanaes HR, Donath K, and Bang G. Titanium implant insertion into dog alveolar ridges augmented by allogenic materials. Clin Oral Implant Res 1994(5): 213–219.

53. Caplanis N, Sigurdsson TJ, Rohrer MD, and Wikesjo UME. Effect of allogeneic, freeze-dried, demineralized bone matrix on guided bone regeneration in supra-alveolar peri-implant defects in dogs. J Oral Maxillofac Implants 1997(12): 634–642.

54. Marthy S and Richter M. Human immunodeficiency virus activity in rib allografts. J Oral Maxillofac Surg 1998(56): 474–476.

55. Frame JW. HA as a biomaterial for alveolar ridge augmentation. Int J Oral Maxillofac Surg 1987(16): 642–655.

56. White E and Shors EC. Biomaterial aspects of Interpore-200 porous hydroxy-apatite. Dent Clin North Am 1986(30): 49–67.

57. Hislop WS, Finlay PM, and Moos KF. Preliminary study into the uses of anorganic bone in oral and maxillofacial surgery. Br J Oral Maxillofac Surg 1993(31): 149–153.

58. Isaksson S, Alberius P, and Klinge B. Influence of three alloplastic materials on calvarial bone healing. Int J Oral Maxillofac Surg 1993(22): 375–381.

59. McCarthy M. Doubt cast on prion infectivity. Lancet 1997(349): 185.

60. Will RG, Ironside JW, and Zeibler M. A new variant of Creutzfeld-Jakob disease in the UK. Lancet 1996(347): 921–925.

61. Morris K, WHO reconsiders risks from Creutzfeld-Jakob disease, Lancet 1997(349): 1001.

62. Ironside JW and Bell JE. The 'high-risk' neuropathology of CJD. Neuropath Appl Neurobiol 1996(22): 388–393

63. Hill AF, Zeidler, Ironside JW, and Collinge J. Diagnosis of new variant CJD by tonsil biopsy. Lancet 1997(349): 99–100.

64. Ashman A. Use of synthetic bone materials in dentistry. Compend Cont Educ Dent 1984(13): 1020–1034.

65. Meffert RM, Thomas JR, Hamilton KM, and Brownstein CN. Hydroxylapatite as an alloplastic graft in the treatment of human periodontal osseous defects. J Periodontol 1985(56): 63–73.

66. Boyne PJ. Advances in preprosthetic surgery and implantation. Curr Opinion Dent 1991(1): 277–281.

67. Dreesman. Uber Knochenplombierung. Bietr Klin Chir 1892(9): 804.

68. Sottosanti J. Calcium sulfate aided bone regeneration. Periodont Clin Invest 1995(17): 2.

69. Shafer C and App G. The use of plaster of Paris in treating infrabony defects in humans. J Periodontol 1971(42): 685.

70. Jarcho M. Biomaterial aspects of calcium phosphates. Dent Clin North Am 1986(30): 25–47.

71. Foitzik C. Treatment of periodontal defects with pure-phase β-tricalcium phospate implant. ZWR 1999(6): 378.

72. Wilson J, and Low SB. Bioactive ceramics for periodontal treatment: Comparative studies in the Patus monkey. J Appl Biomater 1992(3): 123–129.

73. Greenspan DC. Bioglass bioactivity and clinical use. Presented at the Dental Implant Clinical Research Group Annual Meeting 1995, April 27–29.

74. Fetner AE, Hartigan MS, and Low SB. Periodontal repair using perioglass in non-human primates: Clinical and histological observations. Compend Cont Educ Dent 1995(15): 932–938.

75. Schepers EJG, Ducheyne P, Barbier L, and Schepers S. Bioactive glass particles of narrow size range: A new material for the repair of bone defects. Implant Dent 1993(2): 151–156.

76. Schepers E, De Clercq M, Ducheyne P, and Kempeneers R. Bioactive glass particulate material as a filler for bone lesions. J Oral Rehab 1991(18): 439–452.

77. Yukna RA. Clinical evaluation of coralline calcium carbonate as a bone replacement graft material in human periodontal osseous defects. J Periodontol 1994(65): 177–185.

78. Saitoh H, Takata T, Nikau H, Shintani H, Hyon SH, and Ikada Y. Tissue compatibility of polylactic acids in the skeletal site. J Mat Sci Mat Med 1994(5): 194.

79. Boyne P. Use of HTR in tooth extraction sockets to maintain the alveolar ridge height and increase concentration of alveolar bone matrix. Gen Dent 1995(43): 470–473.

80. Wolff J. Das Gesetz der Transformation der Knochen. Berlin: Verlag August Hirschwald, 1892. Reprinted by Repro Med Schrift 1991(4).

81. Springorum HW, Adler CP, Jäger W, and Ober E. Tier-expeimentelle Untersuchung der Knochenregeneration. Z Orthop 1977(115): 686–693.

82. Ashman A. Clinical applications of synthetic bone in dentistry. Gen Dent 1992(11): 481–487.

83. Boyne PJ. Bone induction and the use of HTR polymer as a vehicle for osseous inductor materials. Compend Cont Educ Dent 1998(10): s337–341.

84. Szabo G et al. HTR polymer and sinus elevation: A human histological evaluation. J Long-Term Effects Med Implants 1992(2): 81–92.

85. Sarnachiaro O et al. Immediate implantation of osseointegrated implants filled with Bioplant HTR into extraction sockets of cynomolgus monkeys (Macaca fascicularis): longitudinal study, J Vet Dent, in press.

86. Roum S et al. Treating fresh extraction sockets with an alloplast prior to implant placement: Clinical and histological case reports. Pract Periodont Aesth Dent, in press.

87. Rosenlicht J. Immediate post-extraction placement of an alloplast and titanium screw implant. Pract Periodont Aesth Dent 1993(5): 53–55.

88. Hurley LA, Stinchfield FE, Bassett CAL, and Lyon WH. The role of soft tissues in osteogenesis. J Bone Joint Surg 1959(41A): 1243–1254.

89. Nyman S, Lyndhe J, Karring T, and Rylander H. New attachment following surgical treatment of human periodontal disease. J Clin Periodontol 1982(9): 290–296.

90. Karring T, Nyman S, Gottlow J, and Laurell I. Development of the biological of guided tissue regeneration—Animal and human studies. Periodontol 2000 1993(1): 26–35.

91. Buser D, Dahlin C, and Schenk RK. Guided Bone Regeneration in Implant Dentistry. Berlin: Quintessence Publications, 1994.

92. Wang HL and Carroll WJ. Using absorbable collagen membranes for guided tissue regeneration, guided bone regeneration and to treat gingival recession. Compendium 2000(21): 399–410.

93. Nevins M, Mellonig J, Clem D, Reiser G, and Buser D. Implants in regenerated bone: Long-term survival. Int J Periodontics 1998(18): 34–45.

94. Ashman A and Gross JS. Synthetic osseous grafting. Biomater Eng Dev, 1998(2): 133–154.

95. Zhao S, Pinholt EM, Madsen JE, and Donath K. Histological evaluation of different biodegradable and non-biodegradable membranes implanted subcutaneously in rats. J Craniomaxillofac Surg 2000;(28): 116–122.

96. Lang NP, Hammede CH, Bragger U, Lehman B, and Nyman SR. Guided tissue regeneration in jawbone defects prior to implant placement. Clin Oral Implant Res 1994(5): 92–97.

97. Bunyaratavay P and Wang HL. Collagen membranes: A review. J Periodontol 2001(2): 215–229.

98. Owens KW and Yukna RA. Collagen membrane resorption in dogs: A comparative study. Implant Dent 2001(10): 49–56.

99. Levander G. A study of bone regeneration. Surg Gynecol Obstet 1938(67): 705–714.

100. Lacroix P. Recent investigations on the growth of bone. Nature 1945(156): 576.

101. Urist MR. Bone: Formation by autoinduction. Science 1965(150): 893–899.

102. Wikesjo U, Hanisch O, and Danesh-Meyer MJ. RhBMP-2 for alveolar bone reconstruction in implant dentistry. Dent News 2000(1): 43–47.

103. Wozney JM. Potential role of bone morphogenetic proteins in periodontal reconstruction. J Periodontol 1995(66): 506–510.

104. John HD and Brachwitz J. Praxiserfahrungen mit dem Platelet Concentrate Collection System (3i Implant Innovations). Impl J 2000(4): 44–48.

105. Boyne PJ. Reconstruction of discontinuity mandibular defects in rhesus monkeys using rhBMP-2. J Oral Maxillofac Surg 1995(53): 92–98.

106. McCarthy JG, Staffenberg DA, Wood RJ, Cutting CB, Gray BH, and Thorne ZH. Introduction of an intraoral bone lengthening device. Plast Reconstr Surg 1995(96): 978.

107. Block MS, Chang A, and Crawford C. Mandibular alveolar ridge augmentation in the dog using distraction osteogenesis. J Oral Maxillofac Surg 1996(54): 309.

108. Lazar F, Hidding J, and Zöller JE. Präimplantologische Distraktionsosteogenese. Impl J 2000(4): 18–26.

109. Hidding J, Lazar F, and Zöller JE. Erste Ergebnisse bei der Distraktionsosteogenese des atrophischen Alveolarkammes. Mund Kiefer Gersischtschir 1999 3(Suppl. 1): 79–83.

110. Spiegelberg F. Distraktionsosteogenese im Oberkieferfrontzahnbereich. Impl J 2000(4): 28–32.

111. Gatti A.M , Zaffe D, and Poli GP. Behavior of tricalcium phosphate and hydroxyapatite granules in sheep bone defects. Biomaterials 1990(11): 513–517.

112. Smiler G. Small-segment symphysis graft: Augmentation of the maxillary anterior ridge. Pract Periodont Aesthet Dent 1996(8): 479–483.

113. Jeovanovic SA ,and Nevins M. Bone formation utilizing titanium reinforced barrier membranes. Int J Periodont Rest Dent 1995(15): 57–69.

114. Von Arx T, Hardt N, and Wallkamm B. The TIME technique: A new method for localized alveolar ridge augmentation prior to placement of dental implants. Int J Oral Maxillofac Implants 1996(11): 387–394.

115. Von Arx T, Wallkamm B, and Hardt N. Localized ridge augmentation using a micro titanium mesh: A report on 27 implants followed from 1 to 3 years after functional loading. Clin Oral Implant Res 1998(9): 123–130.

116. Von Arx T and Kurt B. Implant placement and simultaneous peri-implant bone grafting using a micro titanium mesh for graft stabilization. Int J Periodont Rest Dent 1998(18): 117–127.

117. Boyne PJ, Cole MD, Stringer DE, and Shafquat JP. A technique for osseous restoration of deficient edentulous maxillary ridges. J Oral Maxillofac Surg 1985(43): 87–91.

118. Malchiodi L, Scarano A, Quaranta M, and Piattelli A. Rigid fixation by means of titanium mesh in edentulous ridge expansion for horizontal ridge augmentation in the maxilla. Int J Oral Maxillofac Implants 1998(13): 701–705.

119. Steflik DE, Corpe RS, Young TR, and Buttle K. In vivo evaluation of the biocompatibility of implanted biomaterials: Morphology of the implant-tissue interactions. Implant Dent 1998 7(4): 338–350.

120. Misch CE. Treatment plans for implant dentistry. Dent Today 1993(12): 56–61.

121. Misch CE. Divisions of available bone in implant dentistry. Int J Oral Maxilliofac Implants 1990(7): 9–17.

122. Misch CM and Misch CE. The repair of localized severe ridge defects for implant placement using mandibular bone grafts. Implant Dent 1995(4): 261–267.

Index

Page references in *italics* denote photographs or illustrations.